THE COMPLETE MEDITERRANEAN DIET COOKBOOK 2021

300 Tasty, Healthy, Quick, And Affordable Mediterranean Recipes That Will Reset Your Metabolism And Rebalance Your Eating Plans. Including 30-Day Meal Plan

~ 1 ~

© Copyright 2021 - All rights reserved.

Table of Contents

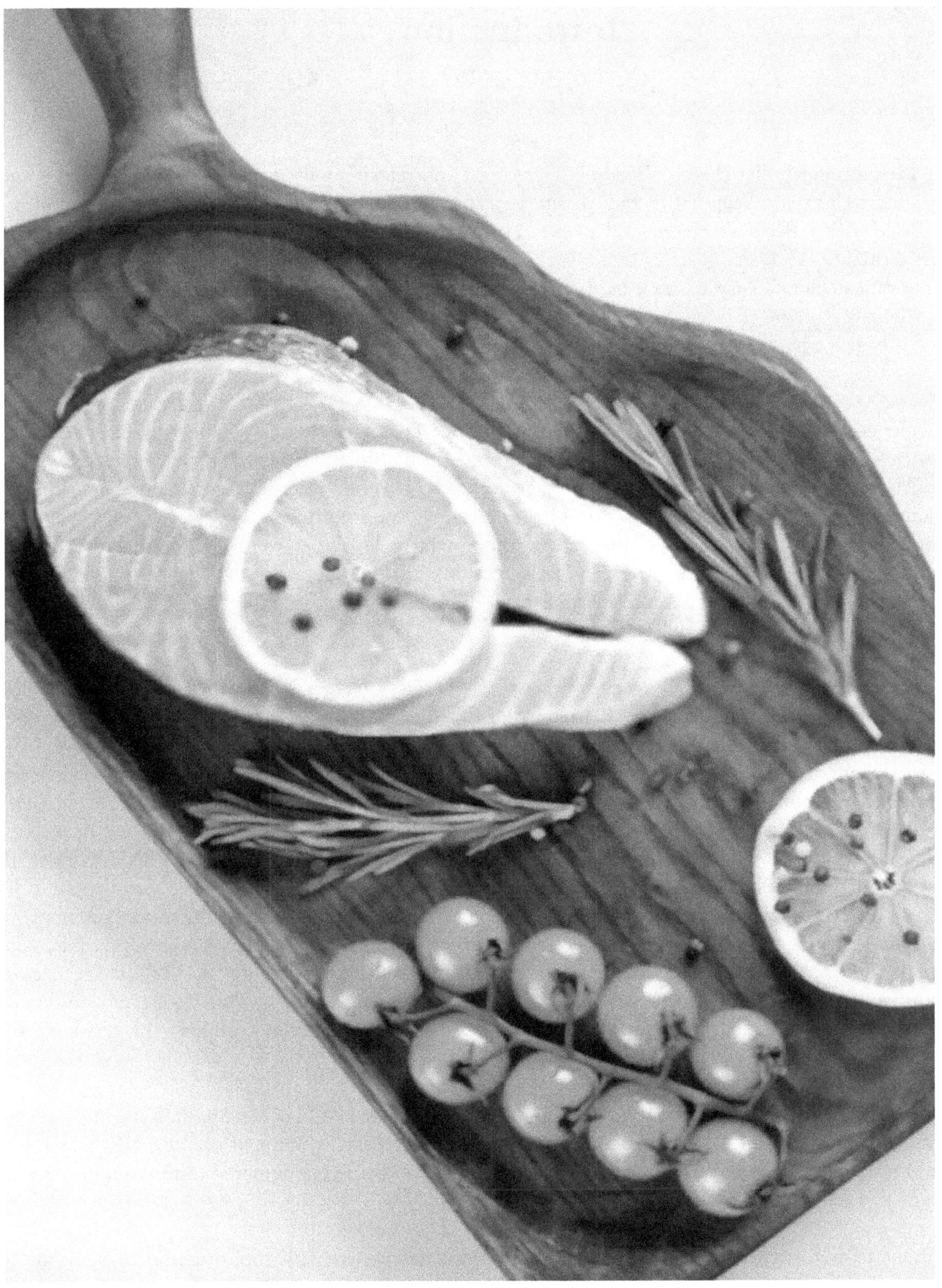

Introduction

The Mediterranean diet claims, shedding a lot of fat and relaxing will keep you healthy. If you want to shed weight and keep it off, the Mediterranean way of life is the solution you've been waiting for. This diet reflects a different way of life. You'll want to hear more about the Mediterranean diet in the long term.

The Mediterranean diet is easy to stick to. It is a basic diet. The Mediterranean diet takes a very direct approach. Italians who are rich live longer than many other people on the planet. The Mediterranean diet has a host of health advantages. Naturally, France and Italy have had a major impact on the Mediterranean diet.

A low incidence of heart disease was found in men who lived in Crete, one of the regions where the Mediterranean diet was first used, according to several medical studies. Fresh fruit, vegetables, olive oil, beans, and herbs are the main ingredients in this diet. Several other studies have found that eating a Mediterranean diet lowers the risk of stroke and hypertension-related mortality.

Studies on the effects of this diet on the skin of those who followed it were also conducted. It was discovered that following this diet helped to avoid skin wrinkling and decreased the chance of skin cancer in those who adopted it. This diet is also helpful to the lungs, as it decreases the risk of clogged arteries, which is something that everyone is afraid of.

The Mediterranean diet is one of my favorites because it is so tasty. Your success when following this diet regimen comes down to truth uncomplicated nature of this diet plan. In all truth, there is no fasting, you must consume it every day. They will certainly try to eliminate their health problems in various ways. It is possible to delight in an extremely healthy and balanced diet regimen with this. This fat-banishing Mediterranean diet regimen can be used by anybody.

The Mediterranean diet is beneficial for your physical health. It's a fantastic way to live. It's a wonderful choice for encouraging weight loss, disease prevention, and good wellbeing.

Another plus is that you will eat your favorite meals while losing weight. Obviously, the more benefits you get from exercising, the more likely you are to continue doing it. If you want to be as safe as possible, you should start with a Mediterranean diet. Sunlight is helpful to one's wellbeing. A healthy lifestyle is beneficial to your well-being. A good life is enhanced by a healthy way of living. The Mediterranean diet is helpful to your health. It is a smart thing to employ a physical strategy to accomplish the objective of getting cured.

The Mediterranean diet is the perfect way to tackle any health issue. When the Mediterranean diet was first discussed publicly in the United States in the 1970s, it referred to a form of cooking that was both healthy and tasty. Today, however, the term refers to a scientific diet that originated in the Mediterranean region many thousands of years ago.

It's important to note that the Mediterranean diet was not developed with the intention of preventing heart disease. It was developed due to the advent of human heart disease. This diet was developed by people who had no idea what heart disease was and didn't feel they were coping with it. At the time, there was no such thing as a diet or food. It was a wonderful and rare way of life. It was set up on very large farms with fields, orchards, vineyards, walnut groves, and olive groves on them. Fresh fruit, nuts, fresh vegetables, herbs, and spices were eaten. They processed their own meat and dairy. They grew their own crops and consumed very little wheat. They ate a wide range of meats, including lamb, goat, turkey, and pork. Basic spices were also used to flavor the food. Since there was plenty of fresh and abundant food, there was no need to make a variety of complex sauces. The more cooked and processed foods were consumed, the more people developed illnesses linked to eating too much of them.

The primitive Mediterranean diet was discovered to be one of the best, if not the best diet that was available, and it was much superior to modern diets.
The Mediterranean diet has been extensively researched. It has been tested from every possible perspective and confirmed to be the safest diet on the planet. The great news is that you won't have to give up any of your favorite foods. It's easy to follow and doesn't necessitate any special cooking methods or nutritionist assistance.

CHAPTER 1:

Basic Principles of The Diet

Learn How to Understand Nutrition Labels

Look for Short Ingredient List: The first ingredient is usually the bulk of the food, which is listed by weight. Put an ingredient back on the shelf if you don't recognize it. Using products containing no more than five ingredients where necessary. Unnecessary extras, such as artificial preservatives, are more likely to blame for the longer ingredient list.

Check Serving Sizes: Frequently, packages contain more than one serving. Think about how much calories and sugar are stored in a single container. Thus, you must first decide the serving amount.

Discover Calorie Counts: It's important to verify the calorie count on the package because it'll help you adhere to the Mediterranean diet schedule.

Avoid fats: It's important to exclude foods that contain entirely hydrogenated or partly hydrogenated oils from your diet.

Check the Percent of Daily Value: The daily value of a packaged item will tell you how many nutrients are in each serving.

Get More of These Nutrients: Look for calcium, iron, fiber, vitamin A, and vitamin C.
The Label Explained
- Serving Information at the Top: This provides the size of one serving and per container.
- Check the total calories per serving and container.
- Limit certain nutrients from your diet.
- Provide yourself with plenty of beneficial nutrients
- Understand the % of daily value section.

Avoid These Foods
- Added Sugar: Ice cream, candy, regular soda, plus many others.
- Refined Oils: Canola oil, cottonseed oil, soybean oil, etc.
- **Trans fats:** Found in various processed foods such as margarine, added sugar, ice cream, candies, table sugar, soda, etc. Added sugars, sugar-sweetened beverages, refined grains, processed meats, and other highly processed foods.
- Processed Meat Products: Hot dogs, processed sausages, bacon
- Refined Grains: Pasta made with refined wheat, white bread

Note If You Are Pregnant: You should avoid some of the oily fish such as swordfish, shark, and tuna because some may contain low levels of toxic heavy metals.
What to Eat Rarely:
- Red meats (Limit to once each week)

Foods You Can Eat

Seafood and Fish: Mussels, clams, crab, prawns, oysters, shrimp, tuna, mackerel, salmon, trout, sardines, anchovies, and more

Poultry: Turkey, duck, chicken, and more

Eggs: Duck, quail, and chicken eggs

Dairy Products: Contain calcium, B12, and Vitamin A: Greek yogurt, regular yogurt, cheese, plus others.

Tubers: Yams, turnips, potatoes, sweet potatoes, etc.

Vegetables: Another excellent choice for fiber and antioxidants: Cucumbers, carrots, Brussels sprouts, tomatoes, onions, broccoli, cauliflower, spinach, kale, eggplant, artichokes, fennel, etc.

Seeds and Nuts: Provide minerals, vitamins, fiber, and protein: Macadamia nuts, cashews, pumpkin seeds, sunflower seeds, hazelnuts, chestnuts, Brazil nuts, walnuts, almonds, pumpkin seeds, sesame, poppy, and more.

Fruits: Excellent vitamin C choices, antioxidants, and fiber: Peaches, bananas, apples, figs, dates, pears, oranges, strawberries, melons, grapes, etc.
Spices and Herbs: Cinnamon, garlic, pepper, nutmeg, rosemary, sage, mint, basil, parsley, etc.

Whole Grains: Whole grain bread and pasta, buckwheat, whole wheat, barley, corn, whole oats, rye, quinoa, bulgur, couscous

Legumes: Provide vitamins, fiber, carbohydrates, and protein: Chickpeas, pulses, beans, lentils, peanuts, peas

Healthy Fats: Avocado oil, avocados, and olives are excellent fats. Olive oil contains monounsaturated fat, which can assist in the removal of 'bad' cholesterol. For some of the world's healthiest populations, the oil has been the conventional fat. Because of the antioxidants and fatty acids in the product, there has been a lot of research showing that it increases the chance of heart disease.
When buying olive oil, bear in mind that it may have been harvested from the olives using chemicals or diluted with cheaper oils like canola or soybean. You should differentiate between refined or light olive oils and regular olive oils. Extra-virgin olive oil is recommended as part of the Mediterranean diet because it has been standardized for purity using natural methods and has superior sensory qualities like taste and scent. The oil contains several phenolic antioxidants, so it's healthy for you.

Beverage Options: Maintaining a healthy body requires lots of water, and the Mediterranean diet plan is no exception. Tea and coffee are appropriate, but fruit juices and sugar-sweetened drinks with high sugar content should be avoided.

White Meats: White meats contains high minerals, protein, and vitamins, but you should remove any visible fat and the skin.

Red Meats: You are allowed red meats, including lamb, pork, and beef, in small quantities. They are rich in minerals, vitamins, and protein—especially iron. Be cautious because they contain more fat—specifically saturated fat—compared to the fat content found in poultry. Don't leave it out entirely; save it for a special dinner or with a stew or casserole.

Potatoes: Potatoes are classified in the tubers class because they are a healthy choice, but how they are cooked will have a significant effect. Potassium, Vitamin B, Vitamin C, and some of the everyday fiber nutrients are all provided. You should bear in mind that they contain a lot of starch, which can easily be transformed to glucose, which can be dangerous and put you at risk for type 2 diabetes. Cook them with less effort, such as baking, boiling, or mashing them without butter.

Desserts and Sweets: Biscuits, cookies, and sweets should only be eaten in small quantities as a special treat. Sugar is not only a source of temptation for type 2 diabetes, but it can also lead to tooth decay. They also produce higher levels of saturated fats as well. You will get some nutritious value, but as a rule, keep your servings small.

What to consume in Moderation: Eggs, poultry, milk, butter, yogurt, and cheese

Improve the Flavor of Foods
When on the diet, you can add flavor and aroma to your food by using her herbs and spices. It will also help you cut back on the amount of salt and fat you use while cooking your meals. Chiles, lavender, tarragon, savory, sumac, and zaatar are some of the spices and herbs that conform to the Mediterranean Diet's requirements.

These are a few more ways you can benefit from spices and herbs:

Anise Benefits: You can aid digestion while also reducing nausea and relieving cramps. After a meal, make some anise tea to help relieve indigestion, bloating, and constipation.

Bay Leaf Benefits: Bay leaves contain magnesium, calcium, potassium, and Vitamins A & C. You are promoting your general health, and it is also proven to be useful in the treatment of migraines.

Basil Benefits: You can get help with digestion, gastric disorders, and flatulence control. You can also greatly manage your diabetes, preserve your heart wellbeing, and reduce depression and anxiety. Try rubbing them onto your scalp after shampooing the next time you have dandruff. The additives assist in the removal of dandruff and dry skin.

Black Pepper Benefits: Pepper aids nutrient absorption in the tissues in the body, stimulates metabolism, and increases digestion. Pepper's key ingredient is a pipeline, which gives it its pungent taste. It can increase fat metabolism by up to 8% for up to many hours after intake. It's used in all of your balanced Mediterranean dishes, as you'll see.

Cayenne Pepper Benefits: Capsaicin, a naturally occurring compound that gives peppers their fiery heat, is the secret ingredient in cayenne. This improves your metabolism for a brief period. Peppers are also high in vitamins, serve as an appetite controller, help with digestion, and are healthy for your heart.

Sweet & Spicy Cloves Benefits: For a spicy taste, add cloves to hot tea. Cloves include antiseptic and germicidal ingredients that can aid with a range of pains, including arthritis, gum and tooth pain, stomach conditions, and infection prevention. Clove oil should be used as an antiseptic for fungal infections, itchy rashes, cuts, and burns. Cloves' fragrance alone can help to stimulate mental imagination.

Ground Chia Seeds Benefits: The seeds can absorb liquid up to 11 times their own weight. Before using them in your recipes, make sure to soak them in plenty of water for at least 5 minutes. Otherwise, you will feel some digestive problems after eating them. Make sure you remain hydrated.

Cumin Benefits: Cumin has been described as spicy, earthy, nutty, and warm in flavor. It's been used as traditional medicine for a long time. It can aid digestion and reduce the risk of foodborne diseases. It will also help you lose weight and regulate your cholesterol and blood sugar levels.

Fennel Benefits: Potassium, phosphorus, vitamin A, calcium, vitamin C, copper, vitamin B6, and magnesium are all nutrients present in fennel. Phosphate and calcium, which are ideal for bone structure—iron and zinc, which are important for collagen production—will boost the bone health. Vitamin C, folate, potassium, and fiber, both of which are contained in fennel, protect your heart health..

Garlic Benefits: Garlic is the best when it comes to reducing blood sugar and helping in weight loss. It assists in appetite management.

Ginger Benefits: Ginger is a diuretic that helps you remove more urine. It's also known for its cholesterol-fighting properties, as well as its ability to improve metabolism and mobility. Ginger can also help fight bloating.

Marjoram Benefits: This is used in the diet to promote healthy digestion, assist with type 2 diabetes management, correct hormone imbalances, and promote restful sleep and a calm mind.

Mint Benefits: Mint helps in the treatment of nasal congestion, nausea, dizziness, and headaches. It helps to improve blood circulation, improves dental health, and helps colic in infants. Mint helps to prevent dandruff and pesky head lice.

Oregano Benefits: Oregano is easy to introduce into your diet, it is rich in antioxidants, and can assist in the fight against bacteria. Oregano is also useful in the treatment of the common cold because it assists in the reduction of infections, the killing of intestinal bacteria, and the relief of menstrual cramps. One major advantage is that it delivers nutrients to the body to aid weight control and digestion.

Parsley Benefits: Using its high amounts of apigenin, a flavonoid, will help the skin, prostate, and digestive system. It has strong antioxidant and inflammatory powers, as well as anti-cancer properties.

Rosemary Benefits: The spice helps increase hair growth, may help relieve pain, eases stress, and also helps reduce joint inflammation.

Sage Benefits: The sage plant's leaves are also used in medicine. It's a perfect way to get rid of diarrhea, abdominal pain or gastritis, heartburn, and gas or flatulence. It may also benefit patients with depression, Alzheimer's disease, memory loss, and several other illnesses.

Tarragon Benefits: The tarragon spice is an excellent choice for maintaining your blood sugar levels, keeping your heart healthy, reduction of inflammation symptoms, improvement of digestive functions, improves central nervous system conditions, and supports healthier eyes.

Thyme Benefits: Thyme is another spice that has been used for protection against the 'Black Death' as well as embalming throughout history. (It's not a pretty dinner suggestion, but it's fascinating nonetheless.) It's also believed to have antibacterial and insecticidal properties. It may be used as an essential oil, a dried herb, or as a fresh herb.

You'll find that the ingredients in your new meal plan have a long list of spices in them. They not only enhance the flavor of your food, but they also improve your wellbeing!

CHAPTER 2:

Breakfast

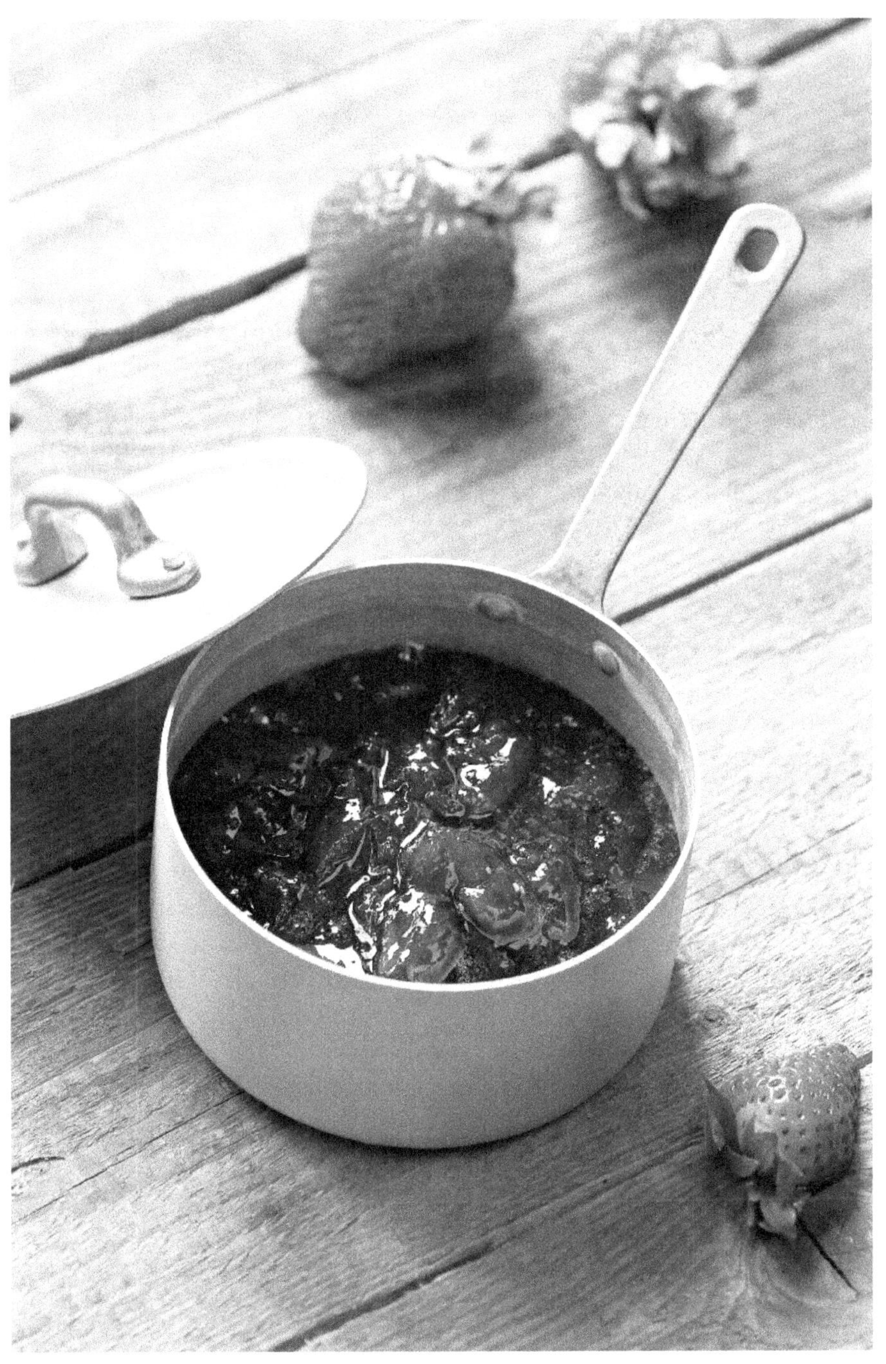

1. Secret Breakfast Sundaes

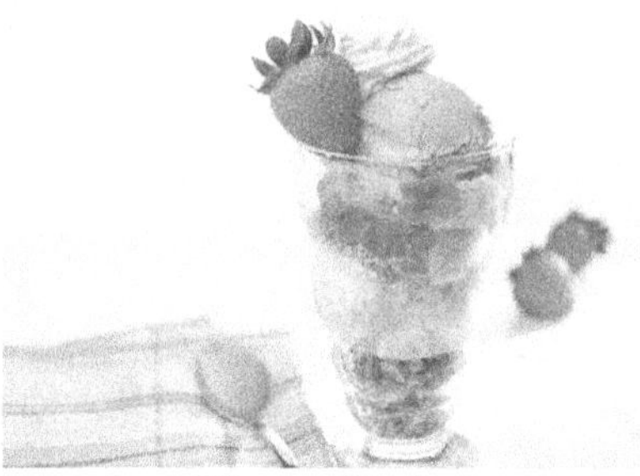

Preparation Time: 5 minutes
Cooking Time: 12 minutes
Servings: 4

Ingredients:

- 6 Slices of Bacon
- 1/2 cup of Heavy Whipping Cream
- 5 tbsp. of Pure Maple Syrup or Pancake Syrup 3 tbsp. of Light Brown Sugar
- 3/4 cup of Granola Cereal 2 cups of Coffee Ice Cream
- 2 cups of Butter Pecan Ice Cream
- 4 Fresh Strawberries

Directions:

1. Preheat your oven to 400 degrees.
2. On a non-stick baking dish, arrange the bacon. Sprinkle half of the brown sugar over the bacon and bake for 6 minutes. Turn the bacon over and top with the remaining brown sugar. Bake for 6 minutes more, or until bacon is dark brown. Remove from the oven and cool on a wire rack. Crumble the bacon and set it aside when it has cooled.
3. In a 2-quart metal mixing dish, whisk together 1 tablespoon maple syrup and 1/2 cup milk with an electric mixer.
4. 4. Divide 2 tablespoons granola into four parfait bottles. Distribute the butter pecan ice cream evenly among the cups and top with the remaining granola. Drizzle the remaining maple syrup over each cup of coffee ice cream equally. Bacon should be sprinkled on top, and strawberries should be placed on top.
5. Serve and Enjoy!

Nutrition:

Calories: 329 kcal
Protein: 7.42 g
Fat: 27.55 g
Carbohydrates: 14.41 g

2. Banana Nut Oatmeal

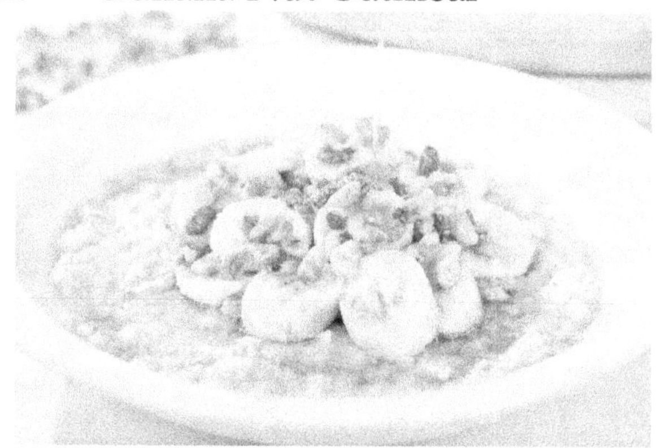

Preparation Time: 5 minutes
Cooking Time: 3 minutes
Servings: 1

Ingredients:

- Peeled Banana
- 1/2 cup of Skim Milk
- 1/4 cup of Quick Cooking Oats
- 3 tbsp. of Honey
- 2 tbsp. of Chopped Walnuts 1 tsp. of Flax Seeds

Directions:

1. 1. In a microwave-safe dish, combine the milk, rice, sugar, walnuts, banana, and flax seeds. Cook for 3 minutes in the oven, then mash the banana with a fork and whisk it into the mixture.
2. Serve and Enjoy!

Nutrition:

Calories: 344 kcal
Protein: 6.8 g
Fat: 4.09 g
Carbohydrates: 75.33 g

3. Greek Frittata w/Zucchini, Tomatoes, Feta, and Herbs

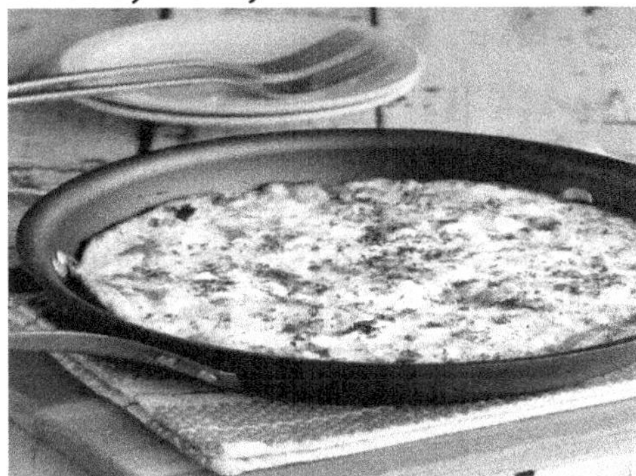

Preparation Time: 10 minutes
Cooking Time: 18 minutes
Servings: 4

Ingredients:

- 6 Eggs
- 15 ounces of Diced Tomatoes 1 Diced Medium Zucchini
- 1 tbsp. of Olive Oil 2 Cloves of Minced Garlic
- 1/2 cup of Mozzarella Cheese 1 tbsp. of Cream
- 1/4 cup of Crumbled Feta Cheese 1/4 tsp. of Oregano
- 1/2 tsp. of Dried Basil
- 1 tsp. of Spike Seasoning Cracked Black Pepper

Directions:

1. Pour your tomatoes into a colander and allow any liquid to flow into the sink. Cut the zucchini's ends and dice it into smaller pieces.
2. Warm up the boiler. Heat olive oil in a frying pan that has been sprayed with cooking spray. Combine the garlic, zucchini, spike seasoning, and dried herb in a mixing bowl. They should be cooked for about 3 minutes. Cook for an extra 3 to 5 minutes after adding the tomatoes. Your tomatoes' liquid should be fully evaporated.
3. Break your eggs in a bowl and beat them well as your vegetables are cooking. Cook for an extra 2 to 3 minutes after pouring the eggs into the pan with your vegetable mixture. The eggs should be only starting to set.
4. Combine half of the feta and mozzarella cheeses in a mixing bowl. Cook for 3 minutes after softly stirring them in. Cook for three more minutes with a lid covering the pan with the rest of the feta and mozzarella cheese sprinkled on top. The eggs should be almost ready and the cheese should be mostly melted.
5. Place under the broiler until the top is finely browned. It shouldn't take more than a few minutes. Keep a close eye on it. If required, rotate the pan to ensure even browning.
6. 6. Garnish with additional fresh herbs if desired. Cut into wedges in the form of a pie.
7. Serve and Enjoy!

Nutrition
Calories: 333 kcal
Protein: 16.77 g
Fat: 26.28 g
Carbohydrates: 7.88 g

4. Greek Yogurt Pancakes

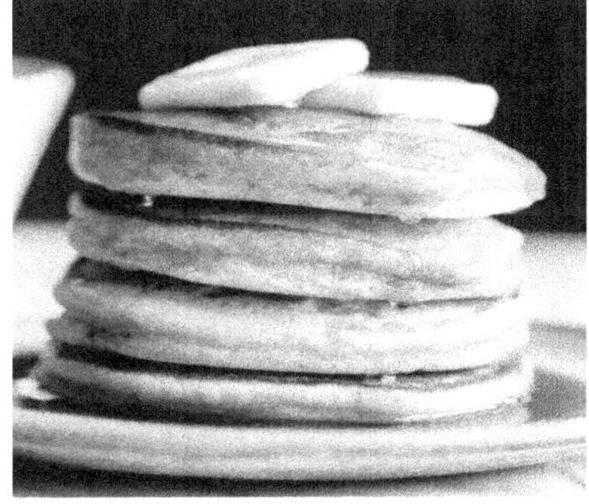

Preparation Time: 20 minutes
Cooking Time: 5 minutes
Servings: 4

Ingredients:

- a cup of Old-Fashioned Oats
- 2 tbsp. of Flax Seeds
- 1 tsp. of Baking Soda
- 1/2 cup of All-Purpose Flour
- 1/4 tsp. of Salt
- 2 cups of Vanilla Greek Yogurt

- 2 tbsp. of Honey or Agave 2 Large Eggs
- 2 tbsp. of Canola Oil Syrup
- Fresh Fruit

Directions:

1. In a blender, blend together the oats, seeds, flour, baking soda, and salt for about 30 seconds.
2. Add in your eggs, yogurt, agave, and oil. Blend until it is smooth. Let your batter stand for approximately 20 minutes to thicken.
3. Heat your skillet over medium heat. Brush your skillet with oil. Spoon your batter 1/4 of a cup at a time into your skillet. Cook your pancakes until the bottoms turn golden brown, and bubbles begin forming on top. It should take about 2 minutes. Turn over your pancakes and cook until the bottoms are golden brown. It should take another 2 minutes.
4. Transfer pancakes to your baking sheet. Keep warm in your oven. Repeat the process until all your batter is cooked.
5. Add on desired syrup and fruit toppings.
6. Serve and Enjoy!

Nutrition
Calories: 172 kcal Protein: 6.62 g
Fat: 4.06 g
Carbohydrates: 37.01 g

5. Mediterranean Tofu Scramble

Preparation Time: 10 minutes
Cooking Time: 10 minutes
Servings: 4

Ingredients:

- 2 tbsp. of Olive Oil 1 Diced Purple Onion
- Two cloves of Minced Garlic
- 1 pound of Extra Firm Tofu
- 1 Diced Medium Red Bell Pepper
- 1 tbsp. of Lemon Juice
- 2 tbsp. of Soy Sauce

- 2 tbsp. of Seasoning
- 1 tsp. of Ground Turmeric
- 1/4 cup of Finely Chopped Fresh Parsley
- Chopped Scallions
- 1/2 tsp. of Red Pepper Flakes Toast
- Hot Sauce Pita Bread Hummus

Directions:

1. Place your big skillet over medium heat and coat the bottom with olive oil. Add the onion to the hot oil and cook until it has softened. It should only take about 5 minutes to complete. Cook for an extra minute after adding the garlic.
2. In a pan, crumble the tofu and add the soy sauce, bell pepper, seasoning, lemon juice, and red pepper flakes. Cook, tossing sometimes with a spatula, until the bell pepper bits are crisp and soft. It should only take about 5 minutes to complete. Remove the pan from the heat and add the scallions and parsley.
3. Serve with pita, toast, hot sauce, and hummus. Enjoy!

Nutrition
Calories: 182 kcal
Protein: 12.7 g
Fat: 11.16 g
Carbohydrates: 10.1 g

6. Greek Yogurt w/Berries & Seeds

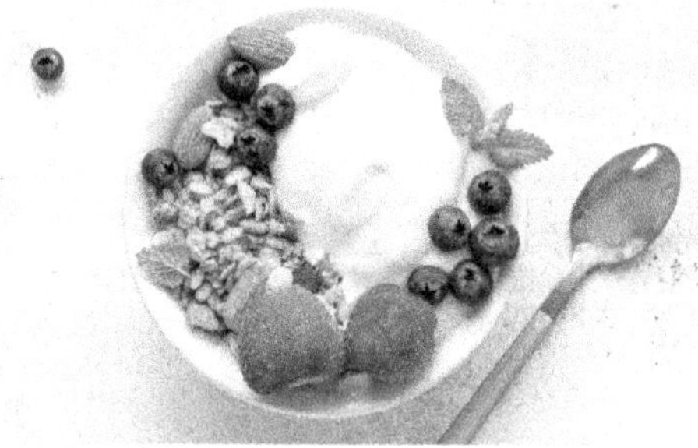

Preparation Time: 3 minutes
Cooking Time: 0 minutes
Servings: 1

Ingredients:

- One handful of Blueberries
- One handful of Raspberries
- 1 tbsp. of Greek Yogurt
- 1 tsp. of Sunflower Seeds
- 1 tsp. of Pumpkin Seeds
- 1 tsp. of Sliced Almonds

Directions:

1. Wash and dry your berries. Place them into a dish.
2. Spoon your Greek yogurt on top and sprinkle it with your seeds and nuts.
3. Serve and Enjoy!

Nutrition

Calories: 127 kcal Protein: 2.28 g

Fat: 3.66 g

Carbohydrates: 23.49 g

7.   Spinach Frittata

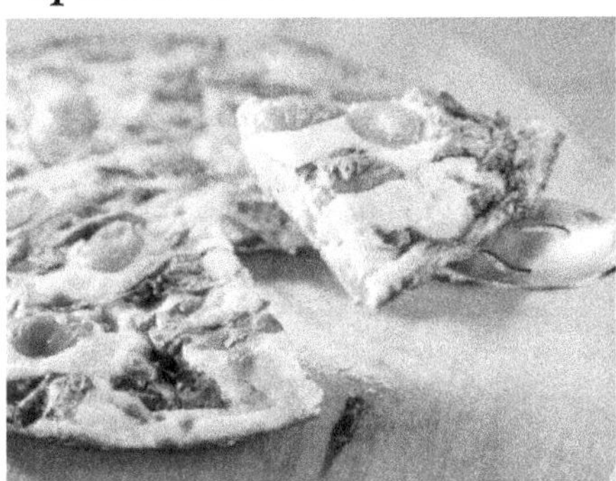

Preparation Time: 15 minutes
Cooking Time: 20 minutes
Servings: 6

Ingredients:

- ¼ cup of kalamata olives, pitted and chopped
- Eight eggs, beaten
- 2 cups of spinach, chopped
- 1 tbsp. of olive oil
- ½ tsp. of chili flakes
- 2 ounces feta cheese, crumbled
- ¼ cup of plain yogurt

Directions:

1. Brush the pan with olive oil. After this, mix up all the remaining ingredients in the mixing bowl, and pour them into the pan. Bake the frittata for 20 minutes at 355 °F. Serve.

Nutrition:

Calories: 145 Protein: 9.6 g

Carbohydrates: 2.3 g Fat: 10.9 g

Fiber: 0.4 g

8.   Mushroom Casserole

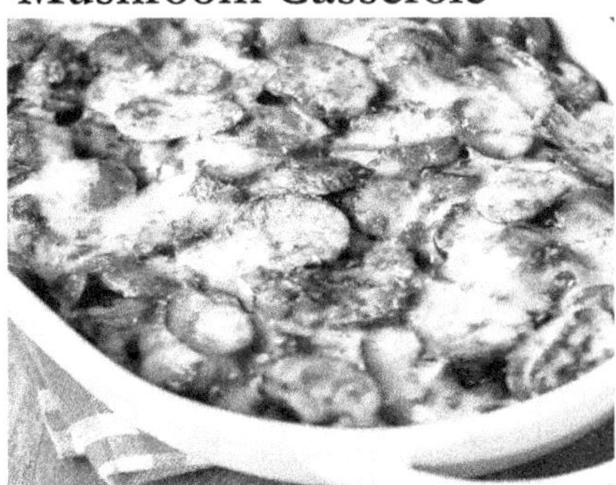

Preparation Time: 15 minutes
Cooking Time: 60 minutes
Servings: 4

Ingredients:

- Two eggs, beaten
- 1 cup of mushrooms, sliced
- Two shallots, chopped
- 1 tsp. of marjoram, dried
- ½ cup of artichoke hearts, chopped
- 3 ounces cheddar cheese, shredded
- ½ cup of plain yogurt

Directions:

1. In a casserole mold, combine all ingredients and cover with aluminum foil.
2. Bake the casserole for 60 minutes at 355 °F.

Nutrition:

Calories: 156

Protein: 11.2 g

Carbohydrates: 6.2 g

Fat: 9.7 g

Fiber: 1.3 g

9.   Vanilla Pancakes

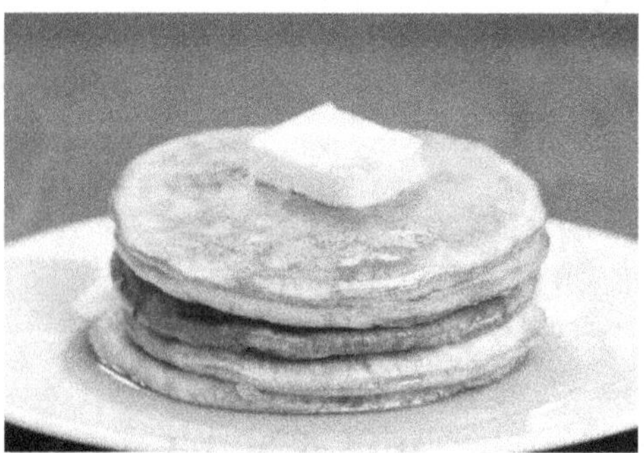

Preparation Time: 15 minutes
Cooking Time: 5 minutes
Servings: 2

Ingredients:

- 6 ounces plain yogurt
- ½ cup of whole-grain flour
- One egg, beaten
- 1 tsp. of vanilla extract
- 1 tsp. of baking powder

Directions:

1. A nonstick skillet should be well heated. Meanwhile, combine all ingredients in a large mixing bowl.
2. In the shape of pancakes, pour the mixture into the skillet.
3. Cook them for 1 minute per side. Serve.

Nutrition:
Calories: 202
Protein: 11.7 g
Carbohydrates: 29.4 g
Fat: 3.8 g
Fiber: 3.7 g

10.   Baked Eggs with Parsley

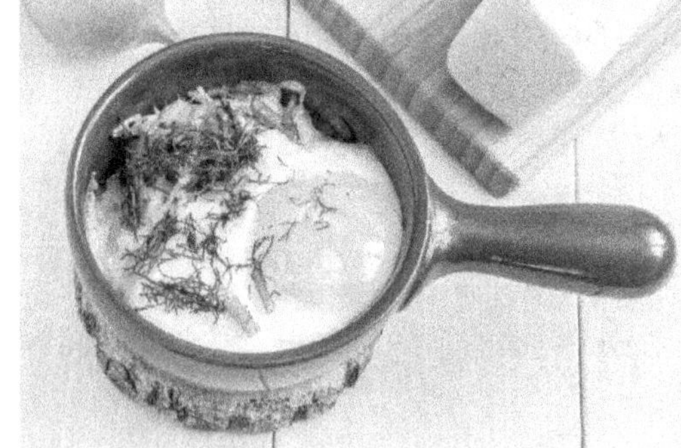

Preparation Time: 15 minutes
Cooking Time: 20 minutes
Servings: 6
Ingredients:

- Two green bell peppers, chopped
- 3 tbsp. of olive oil
- One yellow onion, chopped
- 1 tsp. of sweet paprika
- Six tomatoes, chopped
- Six eggs
- ¼ cup of parsley, chopped

Directions:

1. Warm the oil in a pan over medium heat, then add all of the ingredients except the eggs and roast for 5 minutes.
2. Crack the eggs and stir the vegetables thoroughly.
3. Bake the eggs for 15 minutes in a preheated oven at 360°F.

Nutrition:
Calories: 167
Protein: 3 g
Carbohydrates: 10.2 g
Fat: 11.8 g
Fiber: 2.6 g

11.   Yogurt with Dates

Preparation Time: 10 minutes
Cooking Time: 0 minutes
Servings: 4

Ingredients:

- Five dates, pitted, chopped
- 2 cups of plain yogurt
- ½ tsp. of vanilla extract
- Four pecans, chopped

Directions:

1. In a blender, combine all ingredients and mix until smooth.
2. Pour it into the serving cups.

Nutrition:
Calories: 215
Protein: 8.7 g
Carbohydrates: 18.5 g
Fat: 11.5 g
Fiber: 2.3 g

12.   Mini Frittatas

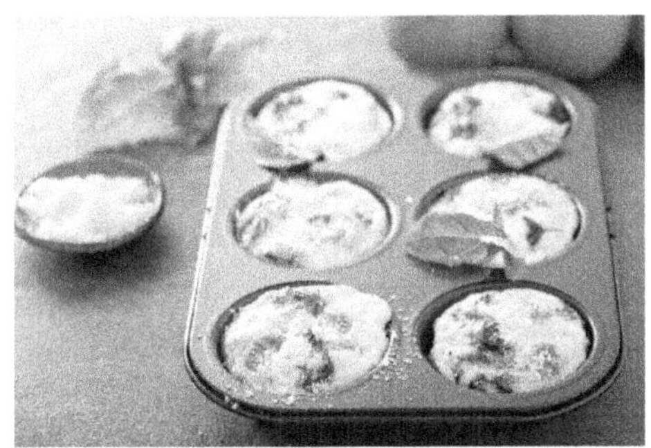

Preparation Time: 5 Minutes
Cooking Time: 15 Minutes
Servings: 12
Ingredients:

- One yellow onion, chopped
- 1 cup parmesan, grated
- One yellow bell pepper, chopped
- One red bell pepper, chopped
- One zucchini, chopped
- Salt and black pepper to the taste
- Eight eggs whisked
- A drizzle of olive oil
- Two tbsp. chives, chopped

Directions:

1. Heat the oil in a skillet over medium-high heat, then add the onion, zucchini, and the remaining ingredients (except the eggs and chives) and cook for 5 minutes, stirring frequently.
2. Spread this mixture in the bottom of a muffin tray, add the egg mixture on top, season with salt, pepper, and chives, and bake for 10 minutes at 350 degrees F.
3. Serve the mini frittatas for breakfast right away.

Nutrition:
Calories 55 Fat 3g
Fiber 0.7g Carbs 3.2g Protein 4.2g

13.   Berry Oats

Preparation Time: 5 Minutes
Cooking Time: 0 Minutes
Servings: 2

Ingredients:

- ½ cup rolled oats
- 1 cup almond milk
- ¼ cup chia seeds
- A pinch of cinnamon powder
- Two tsp. honey
- 1 cup berries, pureed
- One tbsp. yogurt

Directions:

1. Combine the oats, milk, and all other ingredients (except the yogurt) in a mixing dish.
2. Toss all together, divide into bowls, top with yogurt, and serve cold for breakfast.

Nutrition:
Calories 420 Fat 30.3g
Fiber 7.2g Carbs 35.3g Protein 6.4g

14.   Sun-Dried Tomatoes Oatmeal

Preparation Time: 10 Minutes
Cooking Time: 25 Minutes
Servings: 4

Ingredients:

- 3 cups of water
- 1 cup almond milk
- One tbsp. olive oil
- 1 cup steel-cut oats
- ¼ cup sun-dried tomatoes, chopped
- A pinch of red pepper flakes

Directions:

1. Combine the water and milk in a pot and bring to a boil over medium heat.
2. Meanwhile, heat the oil in a pan over medium-high heat, add the oats, and cook for 2 minutes before transferring them to the pan with the milk.
3. Stir in the oats, then add the tomatoes and cook for 23 minutes over medium heat.
4. Divide the mix into bowls, sprinkle the red pepper flakes on top, and serve for breakfast.

Nutrition:
Calories 170 Fat 17.8g
Fiber 1.5g
Carbs 3.8g
Protein 1.5g
Quinoa Muffins
Preparation Time: 10 Minutes
Cooking Time: 30 Minutes

Servings: 12

Ingredients:

- 1 cup quinoa, cooked
- Six eggs whisked
- Salt and black pepper to the taste
- 1 cup Swiss cheese, grated
- One small yellow onion, chopped
- 1 cup white mushrooms, sliced
- ½ cup sun-dried tomatoes, chopped

Directions:

1. Whisk together the eggs, salt, pepper, and the remaining ingredients in a mixing bowl.
2. Divide this into a silicone muffin pan, bake at 350 degrees F for 30 minutes, and serve breakfast.

Nutrition:
Calories 123
Fat 5.6 g
Fiber 1.3g
Carbs 10.8g
Protein 7.5 g

15.   Quinoa and Eggs Pan

Preparation Time: 10 Minutes
Cooking Time: 23 Minutes
Servings: 4

Ingredients:

- Four bacon slices, cooked and crumbled
- A drizzle of olive oil
- One small red onion, chopped
- One red bell pepper, chopped
- One sweet potato, grated
- One green bell pepper, chopped
- Two garlic cloves, minced
- 1 cup white mushrooms, sliced
- ½ cup quinoa
- 1 cup chicken stock
- Four eggs, fried
- Salt and black pepper to the taste

Directions:

1. Over medium-low pressure, heat the oil in a pan, then add the onion, garlic, bell peppers, sweet potato, and mushrooms, tossing and sautéing for 5 minutes.
2. Cook for another minute after adding the quinoa.
3. Add the stock, salt, and pepper, stir and cook for 15 minutes.
4. Divide the mix between plates, top each serving with a fried egg, sprinkle some salt, pepper, crumbled bacon, and serve breakfast.

Nutrition:
Calories 304
Fat 14g
Fiber 3.8g
Carbs 27.5g
Protein 17.8g

16.   Stuffed Tomatoes

Preparation Time: 10 Minutes
Cooking Time: 15 Minutes
Servings: 4

Ingredients:

- Two tbsp. olive oil
- Eight tomatoes, insides scooped
- ¼ cup almond milk
- Eight eggs
- ¼ cup parmesan, grated
- Salt and black pepper to the taste
- Four tbsp. rosemary, chopped

Directions:

1. Using the oil, grease a pan and place the tomatoes inside.
2. Crack an egg into each tomato, split the milk and the remaining ingredients, place the pan in the oven, and bake for 15 minutes at 375 degrees F.
3. Serve for breakfast right away.

Nutrition:
Calories 276
Fat 20.3g
Fiber 4.7g
Carbs 13.2g
Protein 13.7g

17.   Scrambled Eggs

Preparation Time: 10 Minutes
Cooking Time: 10 Minutes
Servings: 2

Ingredients:

- One yellow bell pepper, chopped
- Eight cherry tomatoes, cubed
- Two spring onions, chopped
- One tbsp. olive oil
- One tbsp. caper, drained
- Two tbsp. black olives, pitted and sliced
- Four eggs
- A pinch of salt and black pepper
- ¼ tsp. oregano, dried
- One tbsp. parsley, chopped

Directions:

1. Over medium-high heat, heat the oil in a pan, then add the bell pepper and spring onions and cook for 3 minutes.
2. Sauté for another 2 minutes with the onions, capers, and olives added.
3. Scramble the eggs in the pan with salt, pepper, and oregano for another 5 minutes.
4. Divide the scramble between plates, sprinkle the parsley on top, and serve.

Nutrition:
Calories 249
Fat 17 g
Fiber 3.2g
Carbs 13.3g
Protein 13.5 g

18.   Watermelon "Pizza"

Preparation Time: 10 Minutes
Cooking Time: 0 Minutes
Servings: 4

Ingredients:

- One watermelon slice cut 1-inch thick and then from the center cut into four wedges resembling pizza slices
- Six kalamata olives, pitted and sliced
- 1-ounce feta cheese, crumbled
- ½ tbsp. balsamic vinegar
- One tsp. mint, chopped

Directions:

1. Arrange the watermelon "pizza" on a pan, top with the olives and remaining ingredients, and serve immediately for breakfast.

Nutrition:
Calories 90 Fat 3g
Fiber 1g Carbs 14g Protein 2g

19.   Avocado Egg Scramble

Preparation Time: 8 Minutes
Cooking Time: 15 Minutes
Servings: 4

Ingredients:

- Four eggs, beaten
- One white onion, diced
- One tbsp. avocado oil
- One avocado, finely chopped
- ½ tsp. chili flakes
- 1 oz. Cheddar cheese, shredded
- ½ tsp. salt
- One tbsp. fresh parsley

Directions:

1. Fill the skillet with avocado oil and bring to a boil.
2. Then toss in the diced onion and roast until lightly browned.
3. Meanwhile, combine chili flakes, beaten eggs, and salt.
4. Over medium heat, pour the egg mixture over the cooked onion and simmer for 1 minute.
5. After that, using a fork or spatula, scramble the eggs thoroughly. Cook the eggs until they are solid but not overcooked.
6. After this, add chopped avocado and shredded cheese.
7. Transfer the scrambled eggs to the serving plates after thoroughly stirring them.
8. Fresh parsley should be sprinkled over the meal.

Nutrition:
Calories 236
Fat 20.1g

Fiber 4 g
Carbs 7.4g
Protein 8.6g

20. Morning Pizza with Sprouts

Preparation Time: 15 Minutes
Cooking Time: 20 Minutes
Servings: 6

Ingredients:

- ½ cup wheat flour, whole grain
- Two tbsp. butter softened
- ¼ tsp. baking powder
- ¾ tsp. salt
- 5 oz. chicken fillet, boiled
- 2 oz. Cheddar cheese, shredded
- One tsp. tomato sauce
- 1 oz. bean sprouts

Directions:

1. Make the pizza crust: mix up together wheat flour, butter, baking powder, and salt. Knead the soft and non-sticky dough. Add more wheat flour if needed.
2. Leave the dough for 10 minutes to chill.
3. Then place the dough on the baking paper. Cover it with the second baking paper sheet.
4. Roll up the dough with the help of the rolling pin to get the round pizza crust.
5. After this, remove the upper baking paper sheet.
6. Transfer the pizza crust to the tray.
7. Spread the crust with tomato sauce.
8. Then shred the chicken fillet and arrange it over the pizza crust.
9. Add shredded Cheddar cheese.
10. Bake pizza for 20 minutes at 355F.
11. Then top the cooked pizza with bean sprouts and slice it into the servings.

Nutrition:
Calories 157 Fat 8.8g
Fiber 0.3g Carbs 8.4g
Protein 10.5g

21. Banana Quinoa

Preparation Time: 10 Minutes
Cooking Time: 12 Minutes
Servings: 4

Ingredients:

- 1 cup quinoa
- 2 cup milk
- One tsp. vanilla extract
- One tsp. honey
- Two bananas, sliced
- ¼ tsp. ground cinnamon

Directions:

1. Pour milk into the saucepan and add quinoa.
2. Close the lid and cook it over medium heat for 12 minutes or until quinoa will absorb all liquid.
3. Then chill the quinoa for 10-15 minutes and place in the serving mason jars.
4. Add honey, vanilla extract, and ground cinnamon.
5. Stir well.
6. Top quinoa with banana and stir it before serving.

Nutrition:
Calories 279 Fat 5.3g
Fiber 4.6g Carbs 48.4 g Protein 10.7g

22. Avocado Milk Shake

Preparation Time: 10 Minutes
Cooking Time: 0 Minutes
Servings: 3

Ingredients:

- One avocado, peeled, pitted
- Two tbsp. of liquid honey
- ½ tsp. vanilla extract
- ½ cup heavy cream
- 1 cup milk
- 1/3 cup ice cubes

Directions:

1. Chop the avocado and put it in the food processor.
2. Add liquid honey, vanilla extract, and heavy cream, milk, and ice cubes.
3. Blend the mixture until it smooth.
4. Pour the cooked milkshake into the serving glasses.

Nutrition:
Calories 291

Fat 22.1 g
Fiber 4.5g
Carbs 22g
Protein 4.4g

23. Creamy Oatmeal with Figs

Preparation Time: 10 Minutes
Cooking Time: 20 Minutes
Servings: 5

Ingredients:

- 2 cups oatmeal
- 1 ½ cup milk
- One tbsp. butter
- 3 figs, chopped
- One tbsp. honey

Directions:

1. Pour milk into the saucepan.
2. Add oatmeal and close the lid.
3. Cook the oatmeal for 15 minutes over medium-low heat.
4. Then add chopped figs and honey.
5. Add butter and mix up the oatmeal well.
6. Cook it for 5 minutes more.
7. Close the lid and let the cooked breakfast rest for 10 minutes before serving.

Nutrition:
Calories 222
Fat 6g
Fiber 4.4g
Carbs 36.5g
Protein 7.1g

24. Baked Oatmeal with Cinnamon

Preparation Time: 10 Minutes
Cooking Time: 25 Minutes
Servings: 4
Ingredients:

- 1 cup oatmeal
- 1/3 cup milk
- One pear, chopped
- One tsp. vanilla extract
- One tbsp. Splenda
- One tsp. butter
- ½ tsp. ground cinnamon
- One egg, beaten

Directions:

1. The big bowl mixes up together oatmeal, milk, egg, vanilla extract, Splenda, and ground cinnamon.
2. Melt butter and add it to the oatmeal mixture.
3. Then add chopped pear and stir it well.
4. Transfer the oatmeal mixture to the casserole mold and flatten gently. Cover it with foil and secure edges.
5. Bake the oatmeal for 25 minutes at 350F.

Nutrition:
Calories 151
Fat 3.9g
Fiber 3.3g
Carbs 23.6g
Protein 4.9g

25. Almond Chia Porridge

Preparation Time: 10 Minutes
Cooking Time: 30 Minutes
Servings: 4
Ingredients:

- 3 cups organic almond milk
- 1/3 cup chia seeds, dried
- One tsp. vanilla extract
- One tbsp. honey
- ¼ tsp. ground cardamom

Directions:

1. Bring the almond milk to a boil in a saucepan.
2. Then chill the almond milk to room temperature (or appx. For 10-15 minutes).
3. Add vanilla extract, honey, and ground cardamom. Stir well.
4. After this, add chia seeds and stir again.
5. Close the lid and let chia seeds soak the liquid for 20-25 minutes.
6. Transfer the cooked porridge into the serving ramekins.

Nutrition:
Calories 150
Fat 7.3g
Fiber 6.1g
Carbs 18g
Protein 3.7g

~ 27 ~

CHAPTER 3:

Main Dishes

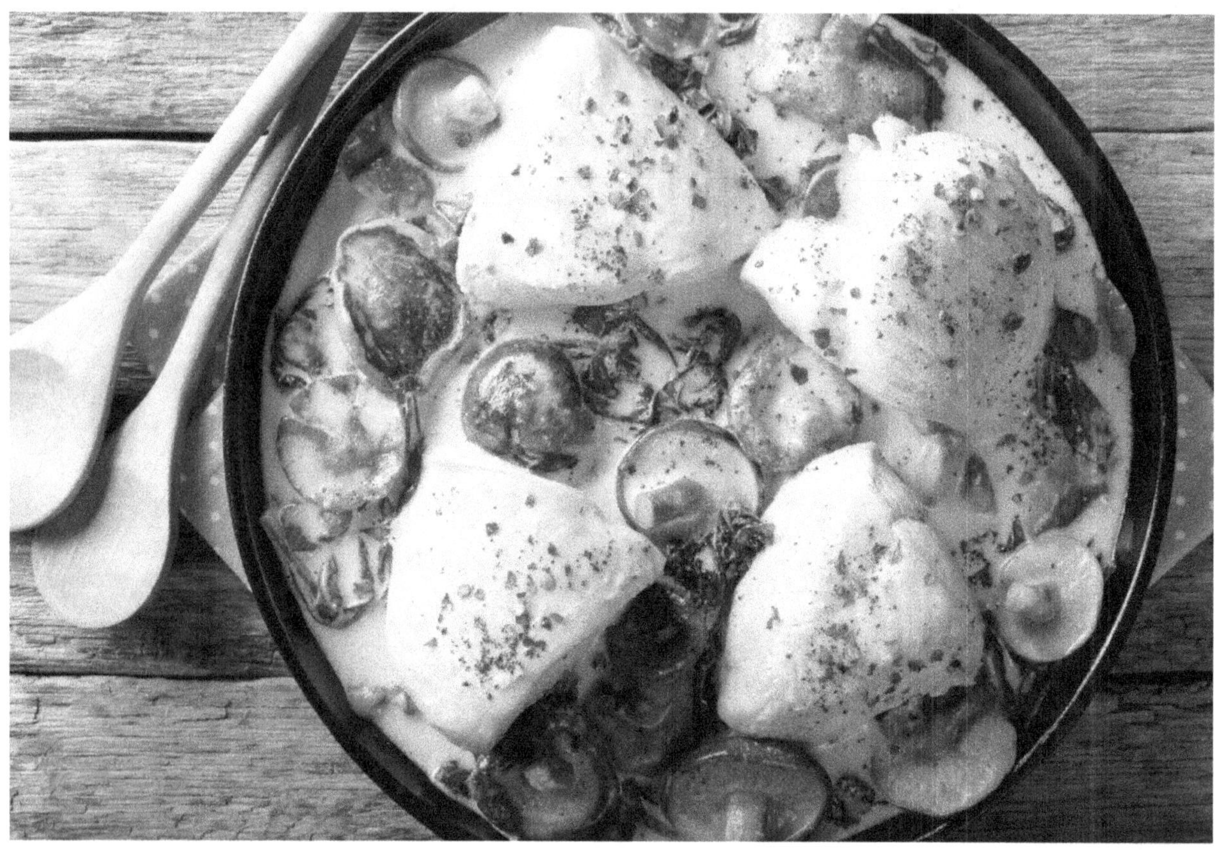

1. Steak with Olives and Mushrooms

Preparation Time: 20 minutes
Cooking Time: 9 minutes
Serving: 6
Ingredients:

- 1 lb. boneless beef sirloin steak
- One large onion, sliced
- 5-6 white button mushrooms
- 1/2 cup green olives, coarsely chopped
- 4 tbsp. extra virgin olive oil

Directions:

1. Heat olive oil set over medium-high heat in a heavy-bottomed skillet. Brown the steaks on both sides then put aside.
2. Gently sauté the onion in the same skillet for 2-3 minutes, stirring rarely. Sauté in the mushrooms and olives.

Nutrition:
Calories: 299
Fat: 56g
Protein: 16g

2. Spicy Mustard Chicken

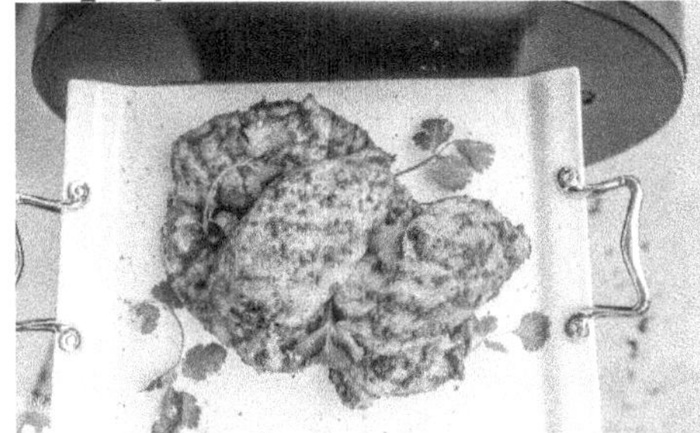

Preparation Time: 32 minutes
Cooking Time: 36 minutes
Serving: 4

Ingredients:

- Four chicken breasts
- Two garlic cloves, crushed
- 1/3 cup chicken broth
- 3 tbsp. Dijon mustard
- 1 tsp. chili powder

Directions:

1. In a small bowl, mix the mustard, chicken broth, garlic, and chili. Marinate the chicken for 30 minutes.
2. Bake in a preheated to 375 F oven for 35 minutes.

Nutrition
Calories 302
Fat 18g
Protein 49g

3. Walnut and Oregano Crusted Chicken

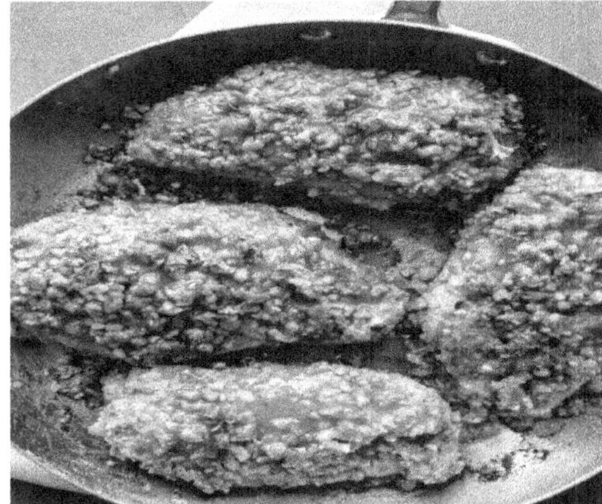

Preparation Time: 36 minutes
Cooking Time: 13 minutes
Serving: 4

Ingredients:

- Four skinless, boneless chicken breasts
- 10-12 fresh oregano leaves
- 1/2 cup walnuts, chopped
- Two garlic cloves, chopped
- Two eggs, beaten

Directions:

1. Blend the garlic, oregano, and walnuts in a food processor until a rough crumb is formed. Place this mixture on a plate.
2. Whisk eggs in a deep bowl. Soak each chicken breast in the beaten egg, and then roll it in the walnut mixture. Place coated chicken on a baking tray and bake at 375 F for 13 minutes on each side.

Nutrition
Calories 304
Fat 54g
Protein 14g

Calories 304
Fat 48g
Protein 13g
Nutrition
Calories: 332 kcalProtein: 16.42 g
Fat: 27.27 g
Carbohydrates: 5.89 g

4. Baked Lemon-Butter Fish

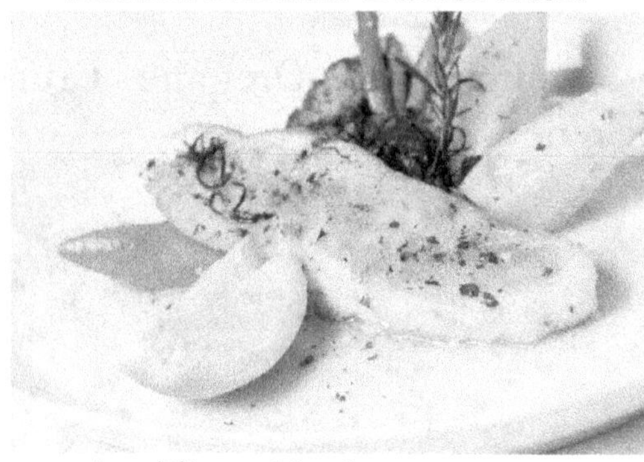

Preparation Time: 10 minutes
Cooking Time: 17 minutes
Serving: 4

Ingredients:

- 4 tbsp. butter, plus more for coating
- 2 (5-ounce) tilapia fillets
- Two garlic cloves, minced
- One lemon, zested and juiced
- 2 tbsp. capers, rinsed and chopped

Direction

1. Preheat the oven to 400°F. Coat an 8-inch baking dish with butter.
2. Pat dries the tilapia with paper towels and season on both sides with pink Himalayan salt and pepper. Place in the greased baking dish.
3. In a medium skillet at medium heat, heat butter. Add the garlic and cook for 3 to 5 minutes, until slightly browned but not burned.
4. Remove the garlic butter from the heat, and mix in the lemon zest and 2 tbsp. of lemon juice.
5. Pour the lemon-butter sauce over the fish, and sprinkle the capers around the baking pan.
6. Bake for 13 minutes and serve.

Nutrition:
Calories: 163 kcal
Protein: 12.01 g
Fat: 12.58 g
Carbohydrates: 1.54 g

5. Fish Taco Bowl

Preparation Time: 10 minutes
Cooking Time: 15 minutes
Serving: 2
Ingredients:

- 2 (5-ounce) tilapia fillets
- 4 tsp. Tajin seasoning salt, divided
- 2 cups pre-sliced coleslaw cabbage mix
- 1 tbsp. Spicy Red Pepper Miso Mayo, plus more for serving
- One avocado, mashed

Direction

1. Preheat the oven to 425°F. Prep baking sheet with silicone baking mat.
2. Rub the tilapia using the olive oil, and then coat it with 2 tsp. of Tajin seasoning salt. Place the fish in the prepared pan.
3. Bake for 15 minutes, or until the fish is opaque when you pierce it with a fork. Put the fish on a cooling rack and let it sit for 4 minutes.
4. Meanwhile, in a medium bowl, gently mix to combine the coleslaw and the mayo sauce. You don't want the cabbage super wet, just enough to dress it. Add the mashed avocado and the remaining 2 tsp. of Tajin seasoning salt to the coleslaw, and season with pink Himalayan salt and pepper. Divide the salad between two bowls.
5. Shred the fish into small pieces, and add it to the bowls.
6. Top the fish with a drizzle of mayo sauce and serve.

Nutrition
Calories: 387 kcal
Protein: 29.01 g
Fat: 26.96 g
Carbohydrates: 10.92 g

6. Scallops with Creamy Bacon Sauce

Preparation Time: 5 minutes
Cooking Time: 20 minutes
Serving: 2

Ingredients:

- Four bacon slices
- 1 cup heavy (whipping) cream
- ¼ cup grated Parmesan cheese
- 1 tbsp. ghee
- Eight large sea scallops rinsed and patted dry

Direction

1. In a medium skillet at medium-high heat, fry bacon on both sides for 8 minutes. Move the bacon to a plate that is lined with paper towels.
2. Lower the heat to medium. Add the cream, butter, and Parmesan cheese to the bacon grease, and season with a pinch of pink Himalayan salt and pepper. Decrease the heat to low and cook, frequently stirring, for 10 minutes.
3. In a separate prepared large skillet over medium-high heat, heat the ghee until sizzling.
4. Season the scallops with pink Himalayan salt and pepper, and add them to the skillet—Cook for just 1 minute per side. Do not crowd the scallops; cook them in two batches if your pan isn't big enough. You want the scallops on either side to be golden.
5. Move the scallops to a paper towel-lined plate.
6. Divide the cream sauce between two plates, crumble the bacon on top of the cream sauce, and top with four scallops. Serve immediately.

Nutrition

Calories 782 Fat 73g Protein 24g

7. Shrimp and Avocado Lettuce Cups

Preparation Time: 10 minutes
Cooking Time: 5 minutes

Serving: 2

Ingredients:

- 1 tbsp. ghee
- ½ pound shrimp
- ½ avocado, sliced
- Four butter lettuce leaves
- 1 tbsp. Spicy Red Pepper Miso Mayo

Direction

1. Preheat medium skillet over medium-high heat, cook the ghee. Add the shrimp and cook. Season with pink Himalayan salt and pepper. Shrimp are cooked when they turn pink and opaque.
2. Season the tomatoes and avocado with pink Himalayan salt and pepper.
3. Divide the lettuce cups between two plates. Fill each cup with shrimp, ½ cup grape tomatoes, and avocado. Drizzle the mayo sauce on top and serve.

Nutrition:
Calories: 203 kcal Protein: 24.61 g
Fat: 8.95 g Carbohydrates: 6.41 g

8. Garlic Butter Shrimp

Preparation Time: 10 minutes
Cooking Time: 15 minutes
Serving: 2

Ingredients:

- 3 tbsp. butter
- ½ pound shrimp
- lemon halved
- Two garlic cloves, crushed
- ¼ tsp. red pepper flakes (optional)

Direction

1. Preheat the oven to 425°F.
2. Place the butter in an 8-inch baking dish and pop it into the oven while preheating until the butter melts.
3. Sprinkle the shrimp with pink Himalayan salt and pepper.
4. Slice one half of the lemon in thin slices, and cut the other half into two wedges.
5. In the baking dish, add the shrimp and garlic to the butter. The shrimp must be in a single layer. Add the lemon slices.

Sprinkle the top of the fish with the red pepper flakes (if using).

6. Bake the shrimp for 15 minutes, stirring halfway through.

7. Remove the shrimp from the oven, and squeeze juice from the two lemon wedges over the dish. Serve hot.

Nutrition:
Calories: 185 kcal
Protein: 15.82 g
Fat: 12.6 g
Carbohydrates: 2.13 g

9. Parmesan-Garlic Salmon with Asparagus

Preparation Time: 10 minutes
Cooking Time: 15 minutes
Serving: 2

Ingredients:

- 2 (6-ounce) salmon fillets, skin on
- ½ pound fresh asparagus ends snapped off
- 2 tbsp. butter
- Two garlic cloves, minced
- ¼ cup grated Parmesan cheese

Direction:

1. Preheat the oven to 400°F. Have a baking sheet prepared with a silicone baking mat.
2. Pat dries the salmon using a paper towel, and seasons both sides with pink Himalayan salt and pepper.
3. Situate the salmon in the middle of the prepared pan, and arrange the asparagus around the salmon.
4. In a small saucepan over medium heat, melt the butter. Add the minced garlic and stir until the garlic just begins to brown about 3 minutes.
5. Drizzle the garlic-butter sauce over the salmon and asparagus, and top both with the Parmesan cheese.
6. Bake until the salmon is cooked and the asparagus is crisp-tender, about 12 minutes. You can switch the oven to broil at the end of cooking time for about 3 minutes to get a nice char on the asparagus.

7. Serve hot.

Nutrition:
Calories: 572 kcal
Protein: 71.39 g
Fat: 29.65 g
Carbohydrates: 7.14 g

10. Seared-Salmon Shirataki Rice Bowls

Preparation Time: 40 minutes
Cooking Time: 10 minutes
Serving: 4

Ingredients:

- 2 (6-ounce) salmon fillets, skin on
- 4 tbsp. soy sauce (or coconut aminos), divided
- Two small Persian cucumbers or ½ large English cucumber
- 1 (8-ounce) pack Miracle Shirataki Rice
- One avocado, diced

Directions

1. Place the salmon in an 8-inch baking dish, and add 3 tbsp. of soy sauce. Cover and marinate in the refrigerator for 30 minutes.
2. Meanwhile, slice the cucumbers thin, put them in a small bowl, and add the remaining 1 tbsp. of soy sauce. Set aside to marinate.
3. Situate skillet over medium heat, melt the ghee. Add the salmon fillets skin-side down. Pour some of the soy sauce marinade over the salmon, and sear the fish for 3 to 4 minutes on each side.
4. Meanwhile, in a large saucepan, cook the shirataki rice per package instructions:
5. Rinse the shirataki rice in cold water in a colander.
6. In a saucepan filled with boiling water, cook the rice for 2 minutes.
7. Pour the rice into the colander. Dry out the pan.

8. Transfer the rice to the dry pan and dry roast over medium heat until dry and opaque.
9. Season the avocado with pink Himalayan salt and pepper.
10. Place the salmon fillets on a plate, and remove the skin. Cut the salmon into bite-size pieces.
11. Assemble the rice bowls: In two bowls, make a layer of the cooked Miracle Rice. Top each with the cucumbers, avocado, and salmon, and serve.

Nutrition:
Calories: 339 kcal Protein: 35.48 g
Fat: 17.72 g Carbohydrates: 11.27 g

11.   Zoodles with Walnut Pesto
Preparation Time: 10 minutes
Cooking Time: 10 minutes
Serving: 4

Ingredients
- Four medium zucchinis, spiralized
- ¼ cup extra-virgin olive oil, divided
- 1 tsp. minced garlic, divided
- ½ tsp. crushed red pepper
- ¼ tsp. freshly ground black pepper, divided
- ¼ tsp. kosher salt, divided
- 2 tbsp. grated Parmesan cheese, divided
- 1 cup packed fresh basil leaves
- ¾ cup walnut pieces, divided

Directions
1. In a large bowl, stir together the zoodles, 1 tbsp. of the olive oil, ½ tsp. of the minced garlic, red pepper, 1/8 tsp. of the black pepper, and 1/8 tsp. of the salt. Set aside.
2. Heat ½ tbsp. of the oil in a large skillet over medium-high heat. Add half of the zoodles to the skillet and cook for 5 minutes, stirring constantly. Transfer the cooked zoodles into a bowl. Repeat with another ½ tbsp. of the oil and the remaining zoodles. When done, add the cooked zoodles to the bowl.

3. Make the pesto: Prepared the food processor, combine the remaining ½ tsp. of the minced garlic, 1/8 tsp. of the black pepper, and 1/8 tsp. of the salt, 1 tbsp. of the Parmesan, basil leaves, and ¼ cup of the walnuts. Pulse until smooth and then slowly drizzle the remaining 2 tbsp. of the oil into the pesto. Pulse again until well combined.
4. Add the pesto to the zoodles along with the remaining 1 tbsp. of the Parmesan and the remaining ½ cup of the walnuts. Toss to coat well.
5. Serve immediately.

Nutrition
Calories: 166
Fat: 16.0g
Protein: 4.0g
Carbs: 3.0g
Fiber: 2.0g
Sodium: 307mg

12.   Cheesy Sweet Potato Burgers
Preparation Time: 10 minutes
Cooking Time: 20 minutes
Serving: 4

Ingredients
- One large sweet potato (about 8 ounces / 227 g)
- 2 tbsp. extra-virgin olive oil, divided
- 1 cup chopped onion
- One large egg
- One garlic clove
- 1 cup old-fashioned rolled oats
- 1 tbsp. dried oregano
- 1 tbsp. balsamic vinegar
- ¼ tsp. kosher salt
- ½ cup crumbled Gorgonzola cheese

Directions
1. Make puncture to the sweet potato all over using a fork, and microwave on high for 4 to 5 minutes, until softened in the center. Cool slightly before slicing in half.
2. Meanwhile, in a large skillet over medium-high heat, heat 1 tbsp. of the

olive oil. Stir in the onion and sauté for five minutes.

3. Spoon the flesh of a sweet potato out of the skin and put the meat in a food processor. Add the cooked onion, egg, garlic, oats, oregano, vinegar, and salt. Pulse until smooth. Add the cheese and pulse four times to barely combine.

4. Form the mixture into four burgers. Place the burgers on a plate, and press to flatten each to about ¾-inch thick.

5. Wipe out the skillet use a paper towel. Heat the remaining 1 tbsp. of the oil over medium-high heat for about 2 minutes. Add the burgers to the hot oil then reduce the heat to medium—Cook the burgers for 5 minutes per side.

6. Move the burgers to a plate and serve.

Nutrition
Calories: 290 Fat: 12.0g
Protein: 12.0g
Carbs: 43.0g
Fiber: 8.0g
Sodium: 566mg

13.   Eggplant and Zucchini Gratin

Preparation Time: 10 minutes
Cooking Time: 19 minutes
Serving: 6

Ingredients

- Two large zucchinis, finely chopped
- One large eggplant, finely chopped
- ¼ tsp. kosher salt
- ¼ tsp. freshly ground black pepper
- 3 tbsp. extra-virgin olive oil, divided
- ¾ cup unsweetened almond milk
- 1 tbsp. all-purpose flour
- $1/3$ cup plus 2 tbsp. grated Parmesan cheese, divided
- 1 cup chopped tomato
- 1 cup diced fresh Mozzarella
- ¼ cup fresh basil leaves

Directions

1. Preheat the oven and set to 425°F (220°C).

2. In a large bowl, toss together the zucchini, eggplant, salt, and pepper.

3. In a prepared large skillet over medium-high heat, heat 1 tbsp. of the oil. Add half of the veggie mixture to the skillet. Stir for a few times, then cover and cook for about 4 minutes, stirring occasionally. Pour the cooked veggies into a baking dish. Place the skillet back on the heat, add 1 tbsp. of the oil and repeat with the remaining veggies. Add the veggies to the baking dish.

4. For the meantime, heat the milk in the microwave for 1 minute. Set aside.

5. Place a medium saucepan over medium heat. Add the remaining 1 tbsp. of the oil and flour to the saucepan. Whisk together until well blended.

6. Slowly pour the warm milk into the saucepan, whisking the entire time. Continue to whisk frequently until the mixture thickens a bit. Add $1/3$ cup of the Parmesan cheese and whisk until melted. Pour the cheese sauce over the vegetables in the baking dish and mix well.

7. Fold in the tomatoes and Mozzarella cheese—roast in the oven for 10 minutes, or until the gratin is almost set and not runny.

8. Top with the fresh basil leaves and the remaining 2 tbsp. of the Parmesan cheese before serving.

Nutrition
Calories: 122
Fat: 5.0g
Protein: 10.0g
Carbs: 11.0g
Fiber: 4.0g
Sodium: 364mg

14.   Veggie-Stuffed Portobello Mushrooms

Preparation Time: 5 minutes
Cooking Time: 24-25 minutes
Serving: 6

Ingredients

- 3 tbsp. extra-virgin olive oil, divided
- 1 cup diced onion
- Two garlic cloves, minced
- One large zucchini, diced
- 3 cups chopped mushrooms
- 1 cup chopped tomato
- 1 tsp. dried oregano
- ¼ tsp. kosher salt
- ¼ tsp. crushed red pepper
- Six large portobello mushrooms, stems, and gills removed
- Cooking spray
- 4 ounces (113 g) fresh mozzarella cheese, shredded

Directions

1. In a large skillet over medium heat, heat 2 tbsp. of the oil. Add the onion and sauté for 4 minutes. Stir in the garlic and sauté for 1 minute.
2. Stir in the zucchini, mushrooms, tomato, oregano, salt, and red pepper. Cook for 10 minutes, stirring constantly. Remove from the heat.
3. Meanwhile, Set the grill and heat a grill pan over medium-high heat.
4. Brush the remaining 1 tbsp. of the oil over the portobello mushroom caps. Place the mushrooms, bottom-side down, on the grill pan. Cover with a sheet of aluminum foil sprayed with nonstick cooking spray—Cook for 5 minutes.
5. Flip the mushroom caps over, and spoon about ½ cup of the cooked vegetable mixture into each cap. Top each with about 2½ tbsp. of the Mozzarella.
6. Cover and then grill for 4 to 5 minutes, or until the cheese is melted.
7. Using a spatula, transfer the portobello mushrooms to a plate. Let cool for about 5 minutes before serving.

Nutrition

Calories: 111
Fat: 4.0g
Protein: 11.0g

Carbs: 11.0g
Fiber: 4.0g
Sodium: 314mg

15. Brussels sprouts Linguine

Preparation Time: 5 minutes
Cooking Time: 25 minutes
Serving: 4

Ingredients

- 8 ounces (227 g) whole-wheat linguine
- $^1/3$ cup plus 2 tbsp. extra-virgin olive oil, divided
- One medium sweet onion, diced
- 2 to 3 garlic cloves, smashed
- 8 ounces (227 g) Brussels sprouts, chopped
- ½ cup chicken stock
- $^1/3$ cup dry white wine
- ½ cup shredded Parmesan cheese
- One lemon, quartered

Directions

1. Bring a large pot of water let it boil and cook the pasta for about 5 minutes, or until al dente. Drain the pasta and reserve 1 cup of the pasta water. Mix the cooked pasta with 2 tbsp. of the olive oil. Set aside.
2. In a large skillet, heat the remaining $^1/3$ cup of the olive oil over medium heat. Add the onion to the skillet then sauté for about 4 minutes, or until tender. Add the smashed garlic cloves and sauté for 1 minute, or until fragrant.
3. Stir in the Brussels sprouts and cook covered for 10 minutes. Pour in the chicken stock to prevent burning. Once the Brussels sprouts have wilted and are fork-tender, add white wine and cook for about 5 minutes, or until reduced.
4. Add the pasta to the skillet and add the pasta water as needed.
5. Top with the Parmesan cheese and squeeze the lemon over the dish right before eating.

Nutrition

Calories: 502

Fat: 31.0g
Protein: 15.0g
Carbs: 50.0g
Fiber: 9.0g
Sodium: 246mg

16.   Beet and Watercress Salad

Preparation Time: 15 minutes
Cooking Time: 8 minutes
Serving: 4

Ingredients

- 2 pounds (907 g) beets, scrubbed, trimmed, and cut into ¾-inch pieces
- ½ cup water
- 1 tsp. caraway seeds
- ½ tsp. table salt, plus more for seasoning
- 1 cup plain Greek yogurt
- One small garlic clove, minced
- 5 ounces (142 g) watercress, torn into bite-size pieces
- 1 tbsp. extra-virgin olive oil, plus more for drizzling
- 1 tbsp. white wine vinegar, divided
- Black pepper, to taste
- 1 tsp. grated orange zest
- 2 tbsp. orange juice
- ¼ cup coarsely chopped fresh dill
- ¼ cup hazelnuts, toasted, skinned, and chopped
- Coarse sea salt, to taste

Directions

1. Combine the beets, water, caraway seeds, and table salt in the Instant Pot. Set the lid in place. Select the Manual mode and then set the cooking time for 8 minutes on High Pressure. When the timer goes off, do a quick pressure release.
2. Carefully open the lid. Using a slotted spoon, transfer the beets to a plate. Set aside to cool slightly.
3. In a small bowl, combine the yogurt, garlic, and 3 tbsp. of the beet cooking liquid. In a prepared large bowl, toss the watercress with 2 tsp. of the oil and 1 tsp. of the vinegar. Season with table salt and pepper.
4. Spread the yogurt mixture over a serving dish. Arrange the watercress on top of the yogurt mixture, leaving a 1-inch border of the yogurt mixture.
5. Add the beets to a now-empty large bowl and toss with the orange zest and juice, the remaining 2 tsp. of the vinegar and the remaining 1 tsp. of the oil. Season with table salt and pepper.
6. Arrange the beets on top of the watercress mixture. Drizzle with the olive oil and sprinkle with the dill, hazelnuts and sea salt.
7. Serve immediately.

Nutrition
Calories: 240
Fat: 15.0g
 Protein: 9.0g
Carbs: 19.0g
Fiber: 5.0g
Sodium: 440mg

17.   Garlicky Broccoli Rabe

Preparation Time: 10 minutes
Cooking Time: 5-6 minutes
Serving: 4

Ingredients

- 14 ounces (397 g) broccoli rabe, trimmed and cut into 1-inch pieces
- 2 tsp. salt, plus more for seasoning
- Black pepper, to taste
- 2 tbsp. extra-virgin olive oil
- Three garlic cloves, minced
- ¼ tsp. red pepper flakes

Directions

1. Bring 3 quarts of water let it boil in a large saucepan. Add the broccoli rabe and 2 tsp. of the salt to the boiling water and cook for 2 to 3 minutes, or until wilted and tender.
2. Drain the broccoli rabe. Transfer to ice water and let sit until chilled. Drain again and pat dry.

3. In a prepared skillet over medium heat, heat the oil and add the garlic and red pepper flakes. Sauté for about 2 minutes or until the garlic begins to sizzle.
4. Increase the heat to medium-high. Stir in the broccoli rabe and cook for about 1 minute, or until heated through, constantly stirring—season with salt and pepper.
5. Serve immediately.

Nutrition
Calories: 87
Fat: 7.3g
Protein: 3.4g
Carbs: 4.0g
Fiber: 2.9g
Sodium: 1196mg

18. Sautéed Cabbage with Parsley

Preparation Time: 10 minutes
Cooking Time: 12-14 minutes
Serving: 4-6

Ingredients

- One small head of green cabbage (about 1¼ pounds / 567 g), cored and sliced thin
- 2 tbsp. extra-virgin olive oil, divided
- One onion halved and sliced thin
- ¾ tsp. salt, divided
- ¼ tsp. black pepper
- ¼ cup chopped fresh parsley
- 1½ tsp. lemon juice

Directions

1. Place the cabbage in a large bowl with cold water. Let sit for 3 minutes. Drain well.
2. Heat 1 tbsp. of the oil in a skillet set on medium-high heat until shimmering. Add the onion and ¼ tsp. of the salt and cook for 5 to 7 minutes, or until softened and lightly browned. Transfer to a bowl.
3. Heat the remaining 1 tbsp. of the oil in a now-empty skillet over medium-high heat until shimmering. Add the cabbage and sprinkle with the remaining ½ tsp. of the salt and black pepper. Cover and

cook for about 3 minutes, without stirring, or until cabbage is wilted and lightly browned on the bottom.
4. Stir and continue to cook for about 4 minutes, uncovered, or until the cabbage is crisp-tender and lightly browned in places, stirring once halfway through cooking. Off heat, stir in the cooked onion, parsley, and lemon juice.
5. Transfer to a plate and serve.

Nutrition
Calories: 117 Fat: 7.0g
Protein: 2.7g
Carbs: 13.4g
Fiber: 5.1g
Sodium: 472mg

19. Braised Cauliflower with White Wine

Preparation Time: 10 minutes
Cooking Time: 12-16 minutes
Serving: 4-6

Ingredients

- 3 tbsp. plus 1 tsp. extra-virgin olive oil, divided
- Three garlic cloves, minced
- 1/8 tsp. red pepper flakes
- One head cauliflower (2 pounds / 907 g), cored and cut into 1½-inch florets
- ¼ tsp. salt, plus more for seasoning
- Black pepper, to taste
- ¹/3 cup vegetable broth
- ¹/3 cup dry white wine
- 2 tbsp. minced fresh parsley

Directions

1. Combine 1 tsp. of the oil, garlic, and pepper flakes in a small bowl.
2. Heat the remaining 3 tbsp. of the oil in a skillet set on medium-high heat until shimmering. Add the cauliflower and ¼ tsp. of the salt and cook for 7 to 9 minutes, stirring occasionally, or until florets are golden brown.
3. Place the cauliflower to the sides of the skillet. Add the garlic mixture to the center of the skillet. Cook for about 30

seconds, or until fragrant. Stir the garlic mixture into the cauliflower.

4. Pour in the broth and wine and bring to simmer. Reduce the heat to medium-low—cover and cook for 4 to 6 minutes, or until the cauliflower is crisp-tender. Off heat, stir in the parsley, and put seasonings with salt and pepper.

5. Serve immediately.

Nutrition

Calories: 143 Fat: 11.7g Protein: 3.1g
Carbs: 8.7g Fiber: 3.1g Sodium: 263mg

20. Cauliflower Steaks with Arugula

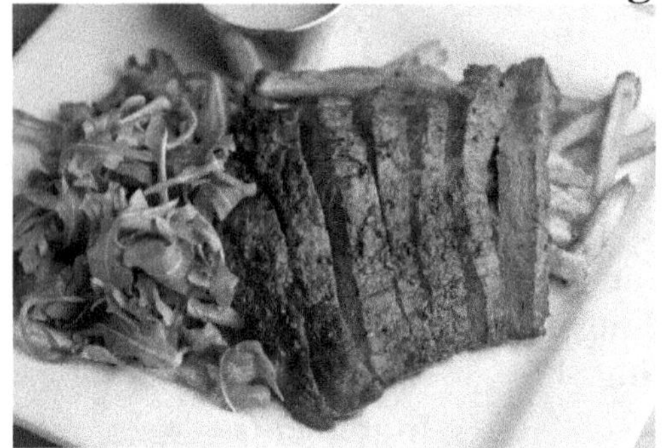

Preparation Time: 5 minutes
Cooking Time: 20 minutes
Serving: 4

Ingredients

Cauliflower:

- One head cauliflower
- Cooking spray
- ½ tsp. garlic powder
- 4 cups arugula

Dressing:

- 1½ tbsp. extra-virgin olive oil
- 1½ tbsp. honey mustard
- 1 tsp. freshly squeezed lemon juice

Directions

1. Preheat the oven set to 425°F (220°C).
2. Remove the leaves from the cauliflower head, and cut it in half lengthwise. Cut 1½-inch-thick steaks from each half.
3. Spritz both sides of each steak with cooking spray and season both sides with garlic powder.

4. Place the cauliflower steaks on a baking sheet, cover with foil, and roast in the oven for 10 minutes.
5. Take the baking sheet from the oven and gently pull back the foil to avoid steam. Flip the steaks, then roast uncovered for 10 minutes more.
6. Meanwhile, make the dressing: Whisk together the olive oil, honey mustard, and lemon juice in a small bowl.
7. When the cauliflower steaks are done, divide into four equal portions. Top each piece with one-quarter of the arugula and dressing.
8. Serve immediately.

Nutrition

Calories: 115
Fat: 6.0g
Protein: 5.0g
Carbs: 14.0g
Fiber: 4.0g
Sodium: 97mg

21. Parmesan Stuffed Zucchini Boats

Preparation Time: 5 minutes
Cooking Time: 15 minutes
Serving: 4

Ingredients

- 1 cup canned low-sodium chickpeas, drained and rinsed
- 1 cup no-sugar-added spaghetti sauce
- 2 zucchinis
- ¼ cup shredded Parmesan cheese

Directions

1. Preheat the oven set to 425°F (220°C).
2. In a medium bowl, stir together the chickpeas and spaghetti sauce.
3. Cut the zucchini in half lengthwise and scrape a spoon gently down each half's length to remove the seeds.
4. Fill each zucchini half with the chickpea sauce and top with one-quarter of the Parmesan cheese.
5. On a baking sheet, put the zucchini

halves and roast in the oven for 15 minutes.

6. Transfer to a plate. Let rest for 5 minutes before serving.

Nutrition

Calories: 139

Fat: 4.0g

Protein: 8.0g

Carbs: 20.0g

Fiber: 5.0g

Sodium: 344mg

22. Baby Kale and Cabbage Salad

Preparation Time: 10 minutes

Cooking Time: 0 minutes

Serving: 6

Ingredients

- Two bunches of baby kale, thinly sliced
- ½ head green savoy cabbage, cored and thinly sliced
- One medium red bell pepper, thinly sliced
- One garlic clove, thinly sliced
- 1 cup toasted peanuts

Dressing:

- Juice of 1 lemon
- ¼ cup apple cider vinegar
- 1 tsp. ground cumin
- ¼ tsp. smoked paprika

Directions

1. In a large mixing bowl, toss together the kale and cabbage.
2. Make the dressing: Mix the cumin, lemon juice, vinegar, and paprika in a small bowl.
3. Pour the dressing over the greens and gently massage with your hands.
4. Add the pepper, garlic, and peanuts to the mixing bowl. Toss to combine.
5. Serve immediately.

Nutrition

Calories: 199 Fat: 12.0g

Protein: 10.0g

Carbs: 17.0g

Fiber: 5.0g

Sodium: 46mg

23. Grilled Romaine Lettuce

Preparation Time: 5 minutes

Cooking Time: 3-5 minutes

Serving: 4

Ingredients

Romaine:

- Two heads of romaine lettuce halved lengthwise
- 2 tbsp. extra-virgin olive oil

Dressing:

- ½ cup unsweetened almond milk
- 1 tbsp. extra-virgin olive oil
- ¼ bunch fresh chives, thinly chopped
- One garlic clove, pressed
- One pinch of red pepper flakes

Directions

1. Heat a grill pan over medium heat.
2. Brush each lettuce half with olive oil. Place the lettuce halves, flat-side down, on the grill. Grill for about 3 to 5 minutes, or until the lettuce slightly wilts and develops light grill marks.
3. Meanwhile, whisk together all the ingredients for the dressing in a small bowl.
4. Drizzle 2 tbsp. of the dressing over each romaine half and serve.

Nutrition

Calories: 126

Fat: 11.0g

Protein: 2.0g

Carbs: 7.0g

Fiber: 1.0g

Sodium: 41mg

24. Mini Crustless Spinach Quiches

Preparation Time: 10 minutes

Cooking Time: 20 minutes

Serving: 6

Ingredients

- 2 tbsp. extra-virgin olive oil
- One onion, finely chopped
- 2 cups baby spinach
- Two garlic cloves, minced
- Eight large eggs, beaten

- ¼ cup unsweetened almond milk
- ½ tsp. sea salt
- ¼ tsp. freshly ground black pepper
- 1 cup shredded Swiss cheese
- Cooking spray

Directions

1. Preheat the oven set at 375°F (190°C). Spritz a 6-cup muffin tin with cooking spray. Set aside.
2. In a prepared large skillet over medium-high heat, heat the olive oil until shimmering. Add the onion and cook for about 4 minutes, or until soft. Add the spinach and cook for about 1 minute, stirring constantly, or until the spinach softens. Add the garlic and sauté for 30 seconds. Remove from the heat and let cool.
3. In a medium bowl, whisk together the eggs, milk, salt, and pepper.
4. Stir the cooled vegetables and the cheese into the egg mixture. Spoon the mixture into the prepared muffin tins—Bake for about 15 minutes, or until the eggs are set.
5. Let rest for 5 minutes before serving.

Nutrition

Calories: 218
Fat: 17.0g
Protein: 14.0g
Carbs: 4.0g
Fiber: 1.0g
Sodium: 237mg

25. Butternut Noodles with Mushrooms

Preparation Time: 10 minutes
Cooking Time: 12 minutes
Serving: 4

Ingredients

- ¼ cup extra-virgin olive oil
- 1 pound (454 g) cremini mushrooms, sliced
- ½ red onion, finely chopped
- 1 tsp. dried thyme
- ½ tsp. sea salt
- 3 garlic cloves, minced
- ½ cup dry white wine
- Pinch of red pepper flakes
- 4 cups butternut noodles
- 4 ounces (113 g) grated Parmesan cheese

Directions

1. In a prepared large skillet over medium-high heat, heat the olive oil until shimmering. Add the mushrooms, onion, thyme, and salt to the skillet. Cook for about 6 minutes, stirring occasionally, or until the mushrooms start to brown. Add the garlic and sauté for 30 seconds. Stir in the white wine and red pepper flakes.
2. Fold in the noodles. Cook for approximately 5 minutes and then stir occasionally, or until the noodles are tender.
3. Serve topped with the grated Parmesan.

Nutrition

Calories: 244 Fat: 14.0g
Protein: 4.0g Carbs: 22.0g Fiber: 4.0g
Sodium: 159mg

26. Potato Tortilla with Leeks and Mushrooms

Preparation Time: 30 minutes
Cooking Time: 50 minutes
Serving: 2

Ingredients

- 1 tbsp. olive oil
- 1 cup thinly sliced leeks
- 4 ounces (113 g) baby bella (cremini) mushrooms, stemmed and sliced
- 1 small potato, peeled and sliced ¼-inch thick
- ½ cup unsweetened almond milk
- 5 large eggs, beaten
- 1 tsp. Dijon mustard
- ½ tsp. salt
- ½ tsp. dried thyme
- Pinch freshly ground black pepper
- 3 ounces (85 g) Gruyere cheese, shredded

Directions

1. Preheat the oven set at 350°F (180°C).
2. In a prepared large sauté pan over medium-high heat, heat the olive oil. Add the leeks, mushrooms, and potato and sauté for about 10 minutes, or until the potato starts to brown.
3. Reduce the heat to medium-low then cover, and cook for an additional 10 minutes, or until the potato begins to soften. Put 1 to 2 tbsp. of water to prevent sticking to the bottom of the pan, if needed.
4. Meanwhile, whisk together the milk, beaten eggs, mustard, salt, thyme, black pepper, and cheese in a medium bowl until combined.
5. When the potatoes are fork-tender, turn off the heat.
6. Transfer the cooked vegetables to an oiled nonstick ovenproof pan and arrange them in a nice layer along the bottom and slightly up the sides of the pan. Pour the milk mixture evenly over the vegetables.
7. Bake in the preheated oven for 25 to 30 minutes or until the eggs are completely set and the top is golden and puffed.
8. Remove from the oven and cool for 5 minutes before cutting and serving.

Nutrition

Calories: 541 Fat: 33.1g
Protein: 32.8g Carbs: 31.0g
Fiber: 4.0g Sodium: 912mg

27. Mushrooms Ragu with Cheesy Polenta

Preparation Time: 20 minutes
Cooking Time: 30 minutes
Serving: 2

Ingredients

- ½ ounce (14 g) dried porcini mushrooms
- 1 pound (454 g) baby bella (cremini) mushrooms, quartered
- 2 tbsp. olive oil
- 1 garlic clove, minced
- 1 large shallot, minced
- 1 tbsp. flour
- 2 tsp. tomato paste
- ½ cup red wine
- 1 cup mushroom stock (or reserved liquid from soaking the porcini mushrooms, if using)
- 1 fresh rosemary sprig
- ½ tsp. dried thyme
- 1½ cups water
- ½ tsp. salt, plus more as needed
- ¹/3 cup instant polenta
- 2 tbsp. grated Parmesan cheese

Directions

1. Immerse the dried porcini mushrooms in 1 cup of hot water for about 15 minutes to soften them. When ready, scoop them out of the water, reserving the soaking liquid. Mince the porcini mushrooms.
2. Heat the olive oil in a large sauté pan over medium-high heat. Add the mushrooms, garlic, and shallot and sauté for 10 minutes, or until the vegetables are beginning to caramelize.
3. Mix in the flour and the tomato paste then cook for an additional 30 seconds. Add the red wine, mushroom stock, rosemary, and thyme. Bring the mixture and let it boil, stirring constantly, or until it has thickened.
4. Reduce the heat and allow simmering for 10 minutes.
5. Meanwhile, bring the water to a boil in a saucepan and sprinkle with the salt.
6. Add the instant polenta and stir quickly while it thickens. Scatter with the grated Parmesan cheese. Taste and season with salt put more as needed. Serve warm.

Nutrition

Calories: 450
Fat: 16.0g
Protein: 14.1g
Carbs: 57.8g
Fiber: 5.0g
Sodium: 165mg

28. Veggie Rice Bowls with Pesto Sauce

Preparation Time: 15 minutes
Cooking Time: 1 minutes
Serving: 2

Ingredients

- 2 cups water
- 1 cup arborio rice, rinsed
- Salt and ground black pepper, to taste
- 2 eggs
- 1 cup broccoli florets
- ½ pound (227 g) Brussels sprouts
- 1 carrot, peeled and chopped
- 1 small beet, peeled and cubed
- ¼ cup pesto sauce
- Lemon wedges, for serving

Directions

1. Combine the water, rice, salt, and pepper in the Instant Pot. Insert a trivet over rice and place a steamer basket on top. Add the eggs, broccoli, Brussels sprouts, carrots, beet cubes, salt, and pepper to the steamer basket.
2. Lock the lid. Select the Manual mode and set the cooking time for 1 minute at High Pressure.
3. When the timer beeps, perform a natural pressure release for 10 minutes, then release any remaining pressure. Carefully open the lid.
4. Remove the steamer basket and trivet from the pot and transfer the eggs to a bowl of ice water. Peel and halve the eggs. Use a fork to fluff the rice.
5. Divide the rice, broccoli, Brussels sprouts, carrot, beet cubes, and eggs into two bowls. Top with a dollop of pesto sauce and serve with the lemon wedges.

Nutrition
Calories: 590
Fat: 34.1g
Protein: 21.9g
Carbs: 50.0g
Fiber: 19.6g
Sodium: 670mg

29. Roasted Cauliflower and Carrots

Preparation Time: 10 minutes
Cooking Time: 30 minutes
Serving: 2

Ingredients

- 4 cups cauliflower florets (about ½ small head)
- 2 medium carrots, peeled, halved, and then sliced into quarters lengthwise
- 2 tbsp. olive oil, divided
- ½ tsp. salt, divided
- ½ tsp. garlic powder, divided
- 2 tsp. za'atar spice mix, divided
- 1 (15-ounce / 425-g) can chickpeas, drained, rinsed, and patted dry
- ¾ cup plain Greek yogurt
- 1 tsp. harissa spice paste, plus additional as needed

Directions

1. Preheat the oven set at 400°F (205°C). Line a sheet pan use foil or parchment paper.
2. Put the cauliflower and carrots in a large bowl. Drizzle with 1 tbsp. of olive oil and sprinkle with ¼ tsp. of salt, ¼ tsp. of garlic powder, and 1 tsp. of za'atar. Toss to combine well.
3. Spread the vegetables onto one half of the prepared sheet pan in a single layer.
4. Put the chickpeas in the same bowl and season with the remaining 1 tbsp. of olive oil, ¼ tsp. of salt, ¼ tsp. of garlic powder, and the remaining 1 tsp. of za'atar. Toss to combine well.
5. Spread the chickpeas onto the other half of the sheet pan.
6. Roast in the preheated oven for 30 minutes, or until the vegetables are crisp-tender. Flip the vegetables halfway through and give the chickpeas a stir so they cook evenly.
7. Meanwhile, whisk the yogurt and harissa together in a small bowl. Taste and add additional harissa as needed.
8. Serve the vegetables and chickpeas with the yogurt mixture on the side.

Nutrition
Calories: 468 Fat: 23.0g
Protein: 18.1g Carbs: 54.1g
Fiber: 13.8g Sodium: 631mg

30.   Sautéed Spinach and Leeks
Preparation Time: 5 minutes
Cooking Time: 8 minutes
Serving: 2

Ingredients

- 3 tbsp. olive oil
- 2 garlic cloves, crushed
- 2 leeks, chopped
- 2 red onions, chopped
- 9 ounces (255 g) fresh spinach
- 1 tsp. kosher salt
- ½ cup crumbled goat cheese

Directions

1. Coat the bottom of Instant Pot using the olive oil.
2. Add the garlic, leek, and onions and stir-fry for about 5 minutes, on Sauté mode.
3. Stir in the spinach. Sprinkle with the salt and sauté for an additional 3 minutes, stirring constantly.
4. Transfer to a plate and scatter with the goat cheese before serving.

Nutrition
Calories: 447 Fat: 31.2g
Protein: 14.6g
Carbs: 28.7g
Fiber: 6.3g
Sodium: 937mg

CHAPTER 4:

Side and Salad Recipes

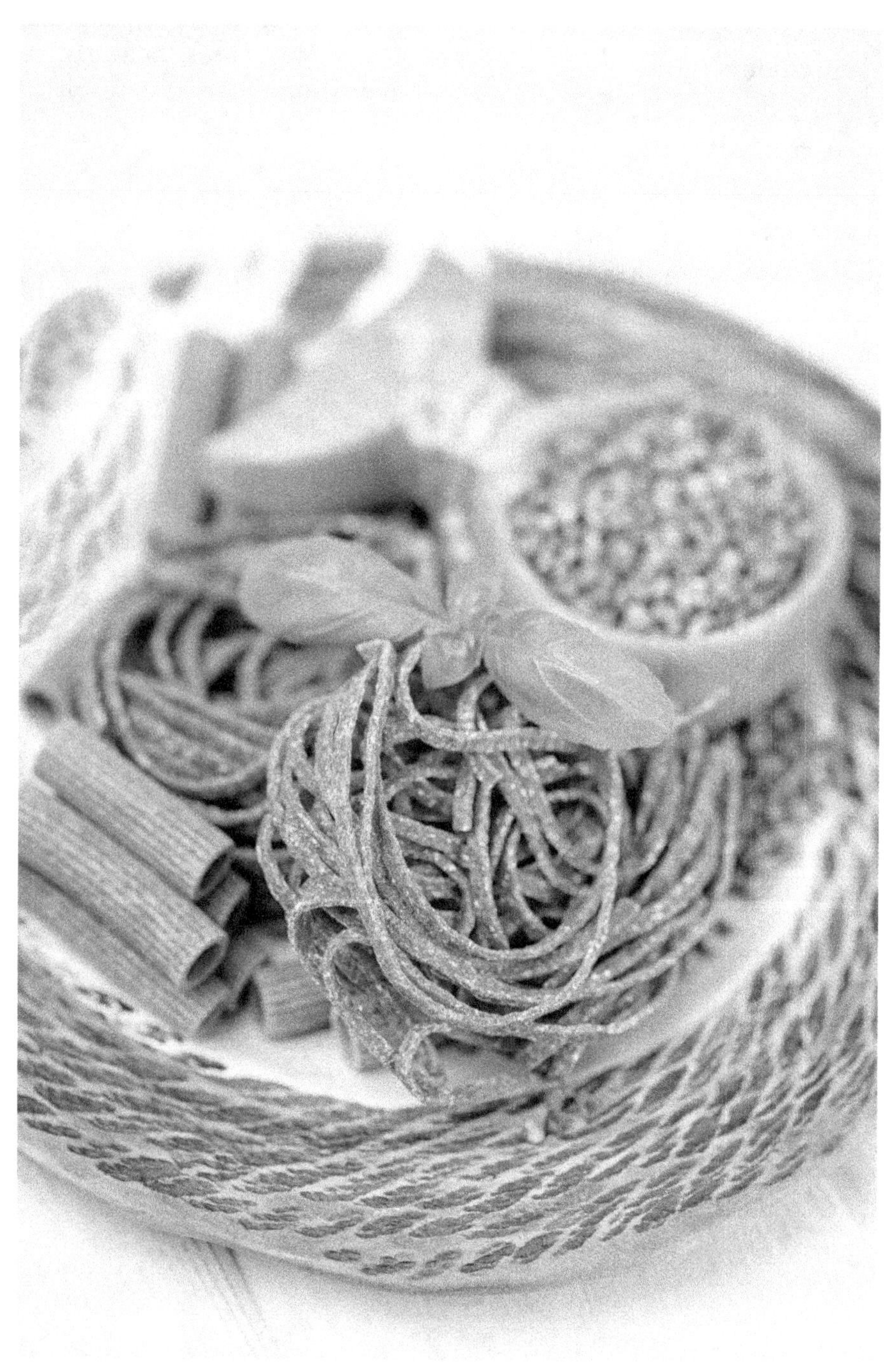

1. Mediterranean Spaghetti

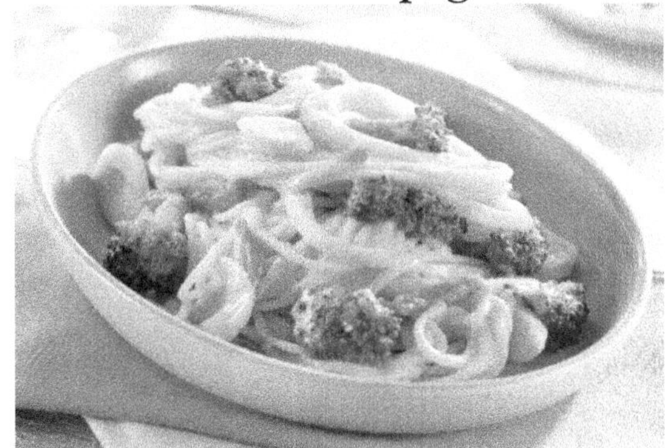

Preparation time: 10 minutes
Cooking time: 10 minutes
Servings: 2

Ingredients:

- 1/3 cup broccoli
- 7 oz. whole grain spaghetti
- 2 oz. Parmesan, shaved
- ½ tsp. ground black pepper
- 1 cup water, for cooking

Directions:

1. Chop the broccoli into the small florets.
2. Pour water in the pan. Bring it to boil.
3. Add broccoli florets and spaghetti.
4. Close the lid and then cook the ingredients for 10 minutes.
5. Then drain water. Add ground black pepper and shaved Parmesan. Shake the spaghetti well.

Nutrition
Calories 430 Fat 8.8g Fiber 9.3g
Carbs 72.4g Protein 23.6 g

2. Hummus Pasta

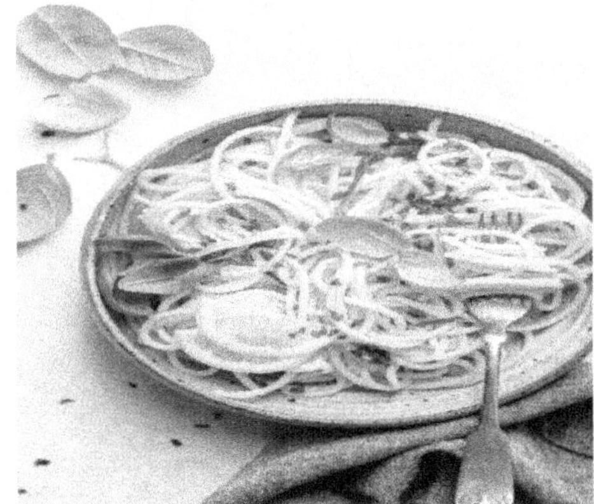

Preparation time: 10 minutes
Cooking time: 15 minutes
Servings: 4

Ingredients:

- 10 oz. soba noodles
- ½ tsp. Italian seasoning
- ¼ tsp. sage
- ¾ tsp. ground coriander
- 4 tsp. hummus
- 1 tsp. butter, softened
- 2 cups water, for cooking

Directions:

1. Pour water in the pan. Bring the liquid to boil.
2. Add soba noodles, sage, and ground coriander.
3. Boil the noodles for 15 minutes over the medium-high heat. The cooked soba noodles should be tender.
4. Then drain water.
5. Mix up together soba noodles, butter, and Italian seasoning.
6. Place the cooked pasta in the bowls and top with hummus.

Nutrition
Calories 256
Fat 2.1g
Fiber 0.3g
Carbs 53.6g
Protein 10.6g

3. Mushroom and Garlic Spaghetti

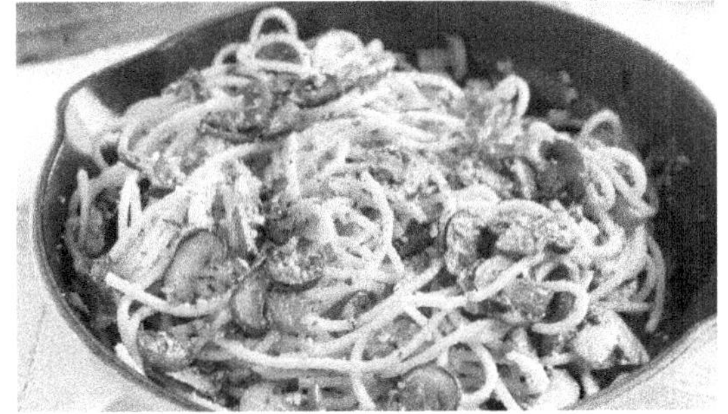

Preparation time: 10 minutes
Cooking time: 20 minutes
Servings: 4

Ingredients:

- ½ cup white mushrooms, chopped
- 3 garlic cloves, diced

- 2 tbsp. sesame oil
- ½ tsp. chili flakes
- 1 tsp. salt
- 1 tsp. dried marjoram
- 10 oz. whole grain buckwheat spaghetti
- 1 cup water, for cooking

Directions:

1. Pour sesame oil in the skillet and heat it up.
2. Add mushrooms and garlic. Mix up well.
3. Sprinkle the vegetables with chili flakes, salt, and dried marjoram.
4. Pour water in the pan and bring to boil.
5. Add buckwheat spaghetti and cook them according to the direction of the manufacturer.
6. Drain water from spaghetti and transfer them in the mushroom mixture.
7. Mix up spaghetti well and cook for 5 minutes over the medium-low heat.

Nutrition
Calories 303
Fat 8.7g
Fiber 5.2g
Carbs 52.4g
Protein 10.4 g

4.   Pasta with Creamy Sauce

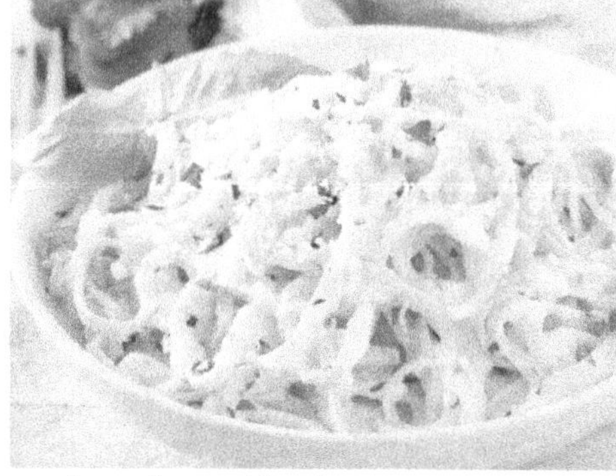

Preparation time: 10 minutes
Cooking time: 7 minutes
Servings: 2

Ingredients:

- 7 oz. quinoa pasta
- 1 tbsp. fresh dill, chopped
- 1 tbsp. fresh cilantro, chopped
- ½ tsp. ground black pepper
- 1 oz. Parmesan, grated
- ½ cup milk
- 1 cup water, for cooking

Directions:

1. Pour water in the pan and bring it to boil.
2. Add quinoa pasta and boil it for 2 minutes. Drain the water.
3. Sprinkle pasta with dill, cilantro, and ground black pepper.
4. Then bring to boil milk and mix it up with Parmesan. Stir well until cheese is melted.
5. Pour the milk sauce over the pasta.

Nutrition
Calories 252
Fat 6.3g
Fiber 2.8g
Carbs 39g
Protein 10.9 g

5.   Feta Macaroni

Preparation time: 15 minutes
Cooking time: 25 minutes
Servings: 4

Ingredients:

- 5 oz. whole grain macaroni
- 4 oz. Feta cheese, crumbled
- 2 eggs, beaten
- ½ tsp. chili pepper
- 1 tsp. almond butter
- 1 cup water, for cooking

Directions:

1. Mix up together water and macaroni and boil according to the directions of the manufacturer.
2. Then drain water.
3. Add almond butter, chili pepper, and Feta cheese. Mix up well.
4. Transfer the mixture in the casserole mold and flatten well.
5. Pour beaten eggs over the macaroni and bake for 10 minutes at 355F.

Nutrition
Calories 262 Fat 11.4g
Fiber 4.2g

Carbs 27.2g
Protein 13.9g

6. Broccoli Puree

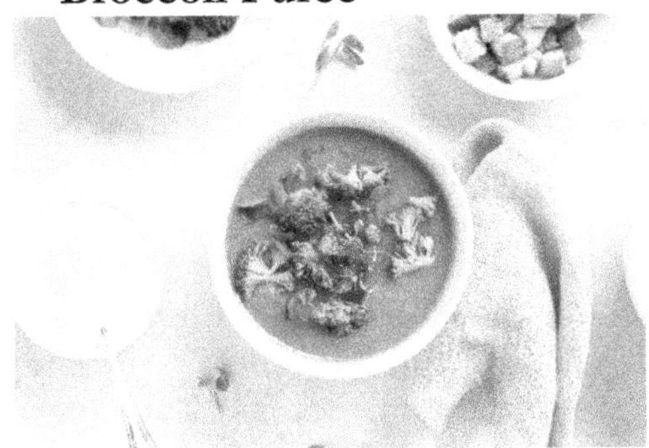

Preparation time: 10 minutes
Cooking time: 15 minutes
Servings: 6

Ingredients:
- 1-pound broccoli, trimmed
- 1 cup chicken stock
- 1 tsp. butter
- 1 tsp. salt

Directions:
1. Line the baking tray with baking paper.
2. Cut the broccoli into the florets and place them on the baking paper.
3. Sprinkle them with salt and bake for 10 minutes at 360F.
4. Meanwhile, pour chicken stock in the pan and bring it to boil.
5. Add baked cauliflower florets and boil them until soft.
6. Then drain ½ part of chicken stock. You can leave less liquid if the broccoli is juicy.
7. Mash the broccoli until you get a soft and fluffy texture.
8. Add butter and mix up with the help of the spoon.

Nutrition
Calories 33 Fat 1g
Fiber 2g Carbs 5.1g Protein 2.2g

7. Margherita Slices

Preparation Time: 5 minutes
Cooking Time: 15 Minutes

Servings: 4

Ingredients:
- 1 Tomato, Cut into 8 Slices
- 1 Clove Garlic, Halved
- 1 tbsp. Olive Oil
- ¼ tsp. Oregano
- 1 Cup Mozzarella, Fresh & Sliced
- ¼ Cup Basil Leaves, Fresh, Tron & Lightly Packed
- Sea Salt & Black Pepper to Taste
- 2 Hoagie Rolls, 6 Inches Each

Directions:
1. Start by heating your oven broiler to high. Your rack should be four inches under the heating element.
2. Place the sliced bread on a rimmed baking sheet. Broil for a minute. Your bread should be toasted lightly. Brush each one down with oil and rub your garlic over each half.
3. Place the bread back on your baking sheet. Distribute the tomato slices on each one, and then sprinkle with oregano and cheese.
4. Bake for one to two minutes, but check it after a minute. Your cheese should be melted.
5. Top with basil and pepper before serving.

Nutrition:
Calories: 297
Protein: 12 g
Fat: 11 g
Carbs: 38 g

8. Vegetable Panini
Preparation Time: 15 minutes
Cooking Time: 25 Minutes
Servings: 4

Ingredients:
- 2 tbsp. Olive Oil, Divided
- ¼ Cup Onion, Diced
- 1 Cup Zucchini, Diced
- 1 ½ Cups Broccoli, Diced
- ¼ tsp. Oregano

- Sea Salt & Black Pepper to Taste
- 12 Oz. Jar Roasted Red Peppers, Drained & Chopped Fine
- 2 tbsp. Parmesan Cheese, Grated
- 1 Cup Mozzarella, Fresh & Sliced
- 2-Foot-Long Whole Grain Italian Loaf, Cut into 4 Pieces

Directions:

1. Heat your oven to 450°F, and then get out a baking sheet. Heat the oven with your baking sheet inside.
2. Get out a bowl and mix your broccoli, zucchini, oregano, pepper, onion and salt with a tbsp. of olive oil.
3. Remove your baking sheet from the oven and coat it in a nonstick cooking spray. Spread the vegetable mixture over it to roast for five minutes. Stir halfway through.
4. Take it from the oven, and add your red pepper, and sprinkle with parmesan cheese. Mix everything together.
5. Get out a panini maker or grill pan, placing it over medium-high heat. Heat up a tbsp. of oil.
6. Spread the bread horizontally on it, but don't cut it all the way through. Fill with the vegetable mix, and then a slice of mozzarella cheese on top.
7. Close the sandwich and cook like you would a normal panini. With a press it should grill for five minutes. For a grill pan cook for two and a half minutes per side. Repeat for the remaining sandwiches.

Nutrition:
Calories: 352
Protein: 16 g
Fat: 15 g
Carbs: 45 g

9.   Baked Tomato

Preparation Time: 7 minutes
Cooking Time: 25 Minutes
Servings: 4

Ingredients:

- Whole grain bread
- Salt and pepper to taste
- 1 tbsp. of finely chopped basil
- 2 cloves of garlic. Finely chopped
- Extra virgin oil
- 2 large tomatoes

Directions:

1. Preheat your oven to 400°F.
2. Use the olive oil to brush the bottom of a baking dish. Set aside.
3. Slice the tomatoes into a thickness of a ½ inch. Lay the tomato pieces into the baking dish that you had prepared earlier. Sprinkle some basil and garlic on top of the tomatoes, season with pepper and salt to taste.
4. Then drizzle the slices of tomatoes with olive oil and then place the baking dish into the oven. Bake for about 20-25 minutes.
5. Remove from the oven, give it a few seconds to cool down and then serve and enjoy.
6. **Tip:** The tomato juice and olive oil at the bottom of the pan can be used as a dipping sauce. So, if you want, you can put it into a small bowl and enjoy it with warm whole grain bread.

Nutrition:
Calories: 342
Protein: 16 g
Fat: 10 g
Carbs: 45 g

10.   Mediterranean Humus Filled Roasted Veggies

Preparation Time: 7 minutes
Cooking Time: 25 Minutes
Servings: 12

Ingredients:

- 6 pitted kalamata olives quartered
- ½ cup (2oz.) of feta cheese
- 1 cup of hummus
- 2 tbsp. of olive oil

- 1 medium red bell pepper
- 1 small zucchini (6 inch)

Directions:

1. Heat a closed medium sized contact grill at 375°F for about 5 minutes.
2. Cut the summer squash and zucchini into half lengthwise. Use a spoon to scoop out the seeds from the two vegetables and discard the seeds.
3. Cut the red bell pepper around the stem and remove the stem and the seeds; cut them into quarters and set aside.
4. Use olive oil to brush the bell pepper, squash and zucchini pieces. Once done, place them on the grill. Do not close the grill.
5. Cook them for 4-6 minutes and turn only once. The vegetables should be tender by the end of the sixth minute. Remove from the grill and let them cool for 2 minutes. Cut the vegetables into 1-inch pieces.
6. Use a spoon to scoop 2 tbsp. of humus onto each piece of vegetable. Light drizzle the vegetables with cheese and top it with one piece of olive. Serve cold or warm.

Nutrition:
Calories: 342
Protein: 10 g
Fat: 15 g
Carbs: 35 g

11.   Goat Cheese Stuffed Tomatoes

Preparation Time: 10 minutes
Cooking Time: 6 minutes
Servings: 4

Ingredients:

- 6-8 arugula leaves
- 3 oz. crumbled feta cheese
- 2 medium ripe tomatoes
- Extra-virgin olive oil to drizzle
- Balsamic vinegar to drizzle
- 1 red onion, very thinly sliced for garnish
- Fresh chopped parsley for garnish
- Salt and freshly ground pepper to taste

Directions:

1. Arrange the arugula leaves in the center of a plate.
2. Remove the tops and the core of the tomatoes. Ideally, you should remove the top first and scoop out the core.
3. Fill the tomatoes with feta cheese. Add salt and pepper, to taste
4. Drizzle with olive oil and balsamic vinegar.
5. Garnish with chopped parsley and red onion.
6. Serve at room temperature.

Nutrition:
Calories: 142
Protein: 7 g
Fat: 13.1 g
Carbs: 7 g

12.   Classic Tabbouleh

Preparation Time: 10 minutes
Cooking Time: 10 minutes
Servings: 4

Ingredients:

- ¾ cup bulgur
- 2 cups freshly chopped parsley
- 1½ cups water
- ½ cup fresh lemon juice
- ½ cup extra-virgin olive oil
- ½ red bell pepper, diced
- 3 ripe plum tomatoes, peeled, seeded, and diced
- 1 large cucumber, peeled, seeded, and diced
- ¾ cup chopped scallions, white and green parts
- ½ green bell pepper, diced
- ½ cup finely chopped fresh mint
- Handful of greens for serving
- Seasoned pita wedges
- Sea salt to taste
- Freshly ground pepper to taste

Directions:

1. Preheat the oven to around 375°F.

2. Take a medium-sized bowl and add the asparagus with 2 tbsp. of salt and olive oil.
3. Take out a baking dish and add the asparagus. Place the tray in the oven then roast for about 10 minutes, or until the asparagus becomes tender.
4. Take out the asparagus and set aside.
5. Use another medium-sized bowl and add garlic, lime juice, orange juice, and remaining 2 tbsp. of olive oil. Whisk all the ingredients together. Add salt and pepper to taste.
6. Take the lettuce and split it into 6 plates. Take out the asparagus and place it on top of the lettuce.
7. Pour the dressing over the asparagus and lettuce salad. Top the salad with basil and pine nuts. Add a small amount of Romano cheese for garnish, if you prefer.
8. In the oven, you can toast the pine nuts as well. Use the method below:
9. Take out a baking tray and line it with a non-stick baking sheet. Add the pine nuts on top.
10. Bake at 375°F for about 5-10 minutes, or until the nuts are lightly browned.
11. Take from the oven then set aside to cool.
12. Add the nuts to the salad as a topping.

Nutrition:
Calories: 177 Protein: 12 g
Fat: 11 g Carbs: 28 g

13. Mediterranean Greens

Preparation Time: 10 minutes
Cooking Time: 0 minutes
Servings: 4

Ingredients:

- 6 cups assorted fresh mixed greens (such as radicchio, arugula, watercress, baby spinach, and romaine)
- 1 small red onion, thinly sliced
- 20 cherry tomatoes, halved
- ¼ cup dried cranberries
- ¼ cup chopped walnuts
- Crumbled feta cheese
- Freshly ground pepper to taste
- 2 tbsp. balsamic vinegar
- 2 cloves fresh garlic, finely minced
- 4 tbsp. extra-virgin olive oil
- 1 tbsp. water
- ½ tsp. crushed dried oregano

Directions:

1. Take out a large salad bowl, combine walnuts, greens, tomatoes, onion, and cranberries. Gently toss.
2. For the dressing, combine water, vinegar, oregano, olive oil, and garlic. Mix the ingredients well. Pour over the salad and lightly toss.
3. Add feta cheese as garnish, if preferred.
4. Add pepper to taste.

Nutrition:
Calories: 140 Protein: 2 g Fat: 12 g
Carbs: 6 g

14. Melon Salad

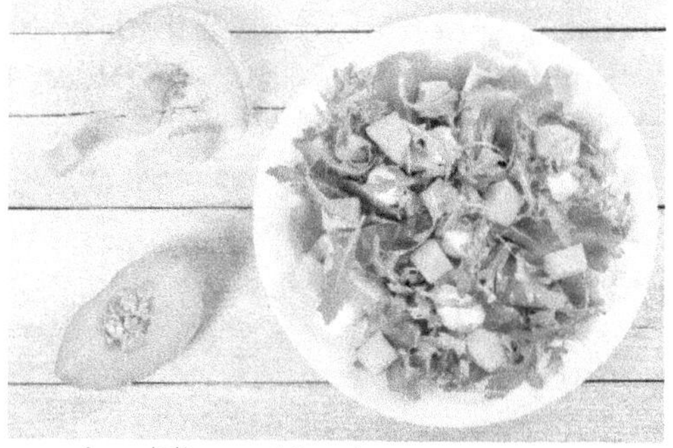

Preparation Time: 10 minutes
Cooking Time: 20 Minutes
Servings: 6

Ingredients:

- ¼ tsp. Sea Salt
- ¼ tsp. Black Pepper
- 1 tbsp. Balsamic Vinegar
- 1 Cantaloupe, Quartered & Seeded
- 12 Watermelon, Small & Seedless
- 2 Cups Mozzarella Balls, Fresh
- 1/3 Cup Basil, Fresh & Torn
- 2 tbsp. Olive Oil

Directions:

1. Get out a melon baller and scoop out

balls of cantaloupe, and the put them in a colander over a serving bowl.

2. Use your melon baller to cut the watermelon as well, and then put them in with your cantaloupe.
3. Allow your fruit to drain for ten minutes, and then refrigerate the juice for another recipe. It can even be added to smoothies.
4. Wipe the bowl dry, and then place your fruit in it.
5. Add in your basil, oil, vinegar, mozzarella and tomatoes before seasoning with salt and pepper.
6. Gently mix and serve immediately or chilled.

Nutrition:
Calories: 218
Protein: 10 g
Fat: 13 g
Carbs: 17 g

15.   Orange Celery Salad

Preparation Time: 5 minutes
Cooking Time: 15 Minutes
Servings: 6

Ingredients:

- 1 tbsp. Lemon Juice, Fresh
- ¼ tsp. Sea Salt, Fine
- ¼ tsp. Black Pepper
- 1 tbsp. Olive Brine
- 1 tbsp. Olive Oil
- ¼ Cup Red Onion, Sliced
- ½ Cup Green Olives
- 2 Oranges, Peeled & Sliced
- 3 Celery Stalks, Sliced Diagonally in ½ Inch Slices

Directions:

1. Put your oranges, olives, onion and celery in a shallow bowl.
2. In a different bowl whisk your oil, olive brine and lemon juice, pour this over your salad.
3. Season with salt and pepper before serving.

Nutrition:

Calories: 65
Protein: 2 g
Fat: 0 g
Carbs: 9 g

16.   Roasted Broccoli Salad

Preparation Time: 30 Minutes
Cooking Time: 30 minutes
Servings: 4

Ingredients:

- 1 lb. Broccoli, Cut into Florets & Stem Sliced
- 3 tbsp. Olive Oil, Divided
- 1 Pint Cherry Tomatoes
- 1 ½ Tsp. Honey, Raw & Divided
- 3 Cups Cubed Bread, Whole Grain
- 1 tbsp. Balsamic Vinegar
- ½ tsp. Black Pepper
- ¼ tsp. Sea Salt, Fine
- Grated Parmesan for Serving

Directions:

1. Preheating your oven set at 450, and then get out a rimmed baking sheet. Place it in the oven to heat up.
2. Drizzle your broccoli with a tbsp. of oil, and toss to coat.
3. Remove the baking sheet form the oven, and spoon the broccoli on it. Leave oil it eh bottom of the bowl and add in your tomatoes, toss to coat, and then toss your tomatoes with a tbsp. of honey. Pour them on the same baking sheet as your broccoli.
4. Roast for fifteen minutes, and stir halfway through your cooking time.
5. Add in your bread, and then roast for three more minutes.
6. Whisk two tbsp. of oil, vinegar, and remaining honey. Season with salt and pepper. Pour this over your broccoli mix to serve.

Nutrition:

Calories: 226
Protein: 7 g
Fat: 12 g
Carbs: 26 g

17.   Tomato Salad

Preparation Time: 5 minutes
Cooking Time: 20 Minutes
Servings: 4

Ingredients:

- 1 Cucumber, Sliced
- ¼ Cup Sun Dried Tomatoes, Chopped
- 1 lb. Tomatoes, Cubed
- ½ Cup Black Olives
- 1 Red Onion, Sliced
- 1 tbsp. Balsamic Vinegar
- ¼ Cup Parsley, Fresh & Chopped
- 2 tbsp. Olive Oil
- Sea Salt & Black Pepper to Taste

Directions:

1. Get out a bowl and combine all of your vegetables together. To make your dressing mix all your seasoning, olive oil and vinegar.
2. Toss with your salad and serve fresh.

Nutrition:
Calories: 126
Protein: 2.1 g
Fat: 9.2 g
Carbs: 11.5 g

18.   Feta Beet Salad

Preparation Time: 5 minutes
Cooking Time: 5 Minutes
Servings: 4

Ingredients:

- 6 Red Beets, Cooked & Peeled
- 3 Oz. Feta Cheese, Cubed
- 2 tbsp. Olive Oil
- 2 tbsp. Balsamic Vinegar

Directions:

1. Combine everything, and then serve.

Nutrition:
Calories: 230
Protein: 7.3 g
Fat: 12 g
Carbs: 26.3 g

19.   Cauliflower & Tomato Salad

Preparation Time: 5 minutes
Cooking Time: 15 Minutes
Servings: 4

Ingredients:

- 1 Head Cauliflower, Chopped
- 2 tbsp. Parsley, Fresh & chopped
- 2 Cups Cherry Tomatoes, Halved
- 2 tbsp. Lemon Juice, Fresh
- 2 tbsp. Pine Nuts
- Sea Salt & Black Pepper to Taste

Directions:

1. Mix your lemon juice, cherry tomatoes, cauliflower, and parsley, and then season. Top with pine nuts, and mix well before serving.

Nutrition:
Calories: 64
Protein: 2.8 g
Fat: 3.3 g
Carbs: 7.9 g

20.   Tuna Salad

Preparation Time: 10 minutes
Cooking Time: 0 minutes
Servings: 2

Ingredients:

- 12 oz. canned tuna in water drained and flaked
- ¼ cup roasted red peppers, chopped
- 2 tbsp. capers, drained
- Eight kalamata olives, pitted and sliced
- 2 tbsp. olive oil
- 1 tbsp. parsley, chopped
- 1 tbsp. lemon juice
- A pinch of salt and black pepper

Directions:

1. In a bowl, combine the tuna with roasted peppers and the rest of the ingredients, toss, divide between plates, and serve breakfast.

Nutrition:
Calories 250
Fat 17.5 g
Fiber 0.6 g

Carbs 2.6 g
Protein 10.4 g

21. Corn and Shrimp Salad

Preparation Time: 10 minutes
Cooking Time: 10 minutes
Servings: 4

Ingredients:

- Four ears of sweet corn, husked
- One avocado, peeled, pitted, and chopped
- ½ cup basil, chopped
- A pinch of salt and black pepper
- 1 lb. shrimp, peeled and deveined
- One and ½ cups cherry tomatoes halved
- ¼ cup olive oil

Directions:

1. Put the corn in a pot, then add water to cover, bring to a boil over medium heat, cook for 6 minutes, drain, cool down, cut corn from the cob, and put it in a bowl.
2. Thread the shrimp onto skewers and brush with some of the oil.
3. In a preheated grill place the skewers, cook over medium heat for 2 minutes on each side, remove skewers, and add over the corn.
4. Put the rest of the ingredients to the bowl, toss, divide between plates, and serve breakfast.

Nutrition:
Calories 316
Fat 22.5 g
Fiber 5.6 g
Carbs 23.6 g
Protein 15.4 g

22. Tahini Spinach

Preparation Time: 5 minutes
Cooking Time: 5 Minutes
Servings: 4

Ingredients:

- 10 Spinach, Chopped
- ½ Cup Water
- 1 tbsp. Tahini
- 2 Cloves Garlic, Minced
- ¼ tsp. Cumin
- ¼ tsp. Paprika
- ¼ tsp. Cayenne Pepper
- 1/3 cup Red Wine Vinegar
- Sea Salt & Black Pepper to Taste

Directions:

1. Add your spinach and water to the saucepan, and then boil it on high heat. Once boiling, reduce to low, and cover. Allow it to cook on simmer for five minutes.
2. Add in your garlic, cumin, cayenne, red wine vinegar, paprika, and tahini. Whisk well, and season with salt and pepper.
3. Drain your spinach and top with tahini sauce to serve.

Nutrition:
Calories: 69
Protein: 5 g
Fat: 3 g
Carbs: 8 g

23. Asparagus Couscous

Preparation Time: 15 minutes
Cooking Time: 30 Minutes
Servings: 6

Ingredients:

- 1 cup Goat Cheese, Garlic & Herb Flavored
- 1 ½ lbs. Asparagus, Trimmed & Chopped into 1 Inch Pieces
- 1 tbsp. Olive Oil
- 1 Clove Garlic, Minced
- ¼ tsp. Black Pepper
- One ¾ Cup Water
- 8 Oz. Whole Wheat Couscous, Uncooked
- ¼ tsp. Sea Salt, Fine

Directions:

1. Preheat your oven set at 425°F, and then put your goat cheese on the counter. It needs to come to room temperature.
2. Get out a bowl and mix your oil, pepper, garlic, and asparagus. Spread the asparagus on a baking sheet and roast for

ten minutes. Make sure to stir at least once.

3. Remove it from the pan, and place your asparagus in a serving bowl.

4. Get out a medium saucepan, and bring your water to a boil. Add in your salt and couscous. Reduce the heat to medium-low, and then cover your saucepan. Cook for twelve minutes. All your water should be absorbed.

5. Pour the couscous in a bowl with asparagus, and ad din your goat cheese. Stir until melted, and serve warm.

Nutrition:
Calories: 263 Protein: 11 g
Fat: 9 g Carbs: 36 g

24. Easy Spaghetti Squash

Preparation Time: 15 minutes
Cooking Time: 25 Minutes
Servings: 4

Ingredients:

- 2 Spring Onions, Chopped Fine
- 3 Cloves Garlic, Minced
- 1 Zucchini, Diced1 Red Bell Pepper, Diced
- 1 tbsp. Italian Seasoning
- 1 Tomato, Small & Chopped Fine
- 1 tbsp. Parsley, Fresh & Chopped
- Pinch Lemon Pepper
- Dash Sea Salt, Fine
- 4 Oz. Feta Cheese, Crumbled
- 3 Italian Sausage Links, Casing Removed
- 2 tbsp. Olive Oil
- 1 Spaghetti Sauce, Halved Lengthwise

Directions:

1. Preheat your oven set at 350°F, and get out a large baking sheet. Coat it with cooking spray, and then put your squash on it with the cut side down.

2. Bake at 350°F for forty-five minutes. It should be tender.

3. Turn the squash over, and bake for five more minutes. Scrape the strands into a larger bowl.

4. Heat a tbsp. of olive oil in a skillet, and then add in your Italian sausage—Cook at eight minutes before removing it and placing it in a bowl.

5. Add another tbsp. of olive oil to the skillet and cook your garlic and onions until softened. That will take five minutes.

6. Throw in your Italian seasoning, red peppers, and zucchini. Cook for another five minutes. Your vegetables should be softened.

7. Mix in your feta cheese and squash, cooking until the cheese has melted.

8. Stir in your sausage, and then season with lemon pepper and salt. Serve with parsley and tomato.

Nutrition:
Calories: 423
Protein: 18 g
Fat: 30 g
Carbs: 22 g

25. Garbanzo Bean Salad

Preparation Time: 10 minutes
Cooking Time: 0 minutes
Servings: 4

Ingredients:

- One and ½ cups cucumber, cubed
- 15 oz. canned garbanzo beans drained and rinsed
- 3 oz. black olives, pitted and sliced
- One tomato, chopped
- ¼ cup red onion, chopped
- 5 cups salad greens
- A pinch of salt and black pepper
- ½ cup feta cheese, crumbled
- 3 tbsp. olive oil
- 1 tbsp. lemon juice
- ¼ cup parsley, chopped

Directions:

1. In a salad bowl, combine the garbanzo beans with the cucumber, tomato, and the rest of the ingredients except the cheese and toss.

2. Divide the mix into small bowls, sprinkle the cheese on top, and serve for breakfast.

Nutrition:
Calories 268
Fat 16.5 g
Fiber 7.6 g
Carbs 36.6 g
Protein 9.4 g

26. Spiced Chickpeas Bowls

Preparation Time: 10 minutes
Cooking Time: 30 minutes
Servings: 4

Ingredients:

- 15 oz. canned chickpeas drained and rinsed
- ¼ tsp. cardamom, ground
- ½ tsp. cinnamon powder
- One and ½ tsp. turmeric powder
- 1 tsp. coriander, ground
- 1 tbsp. olive oil
- A pinch of salt and black pepper
- ¾ cup Greek yogurt
- ½ cup green olives pitted and halved
- ½ cup cherry tomatoes halved
- One cucumber, sliced

Directions:

1. On a lined baking sheet, spread the chickpeas, add the cardamom, cinnamon, turmeric, coriander, the oil, salt, and pepper, toss and bake at 375°F for 30 minutes.
2. In a bowl, combine the roasted chickpeas with the rest of the ingredients, toss, and serve breakfast.

Nutrition:
Calories 519
Fat 34.5 g
Fiber 13.6 g
Carbs 36.6 g
Protein 11.4 g

27. Balsamic Asparagus

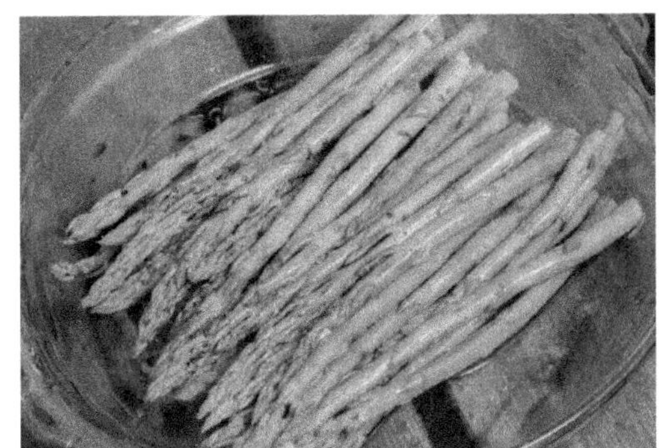

Preparation time: 10 minutes
Cooking time: 15 minutes
Servings: 4

Ingredients:

- 3 tbsp. olive oil
- Three garlic cloves, minced
- 2 tbsp. shallot, chopped
- Salt and black pepper to the taste
- 2 tsp. balsamic vinegar
- One and ½ pound asparagus, trimmed

Directions:

1. Heat a pan with the oil over medium-high heat, add the garlic and the shallot and sauté for 3 minutes.
2. Add the rest of the ingredients, cook for 12 minutes more, divide between plates and serve as a side dish.

Nutrition:
Calories 100
Fat: 10.5 g
Fiber: 1.2 g
Carbs: 2.3 g
Protein: 2.1 g

28. Lime Cucumber Mix

Preparation time: 10 minutes
Cooking time: 0 minutes
Servings: 8

Ingredients:

- Four cucumbers, chopped
- ½ cup green bell pepper, chopped
- One yellow onion, chopped
- One chili pepper, chopped
- One garlic clove, minced
- 1 tsp. parsley, chopped
- 2 tbsp. lime juice

- 1 tbsp. dill, chopped
- Salt and black pepper to the taste
- 1 tbsp. olive oil

Directions:

1. In a prepared large bowl, mix the cucumber with the bell peppers and the rest of the ingredients, toss and serve as a side dish.

Nutrition:
Calories 123
Fat 4.3 g
Fiber 2.3g
Carbs 5.6g
Protein 2 g

29. Walnuts Cucumber Mix

Preparation time: 5 minutes
Cooking time: 0 minutes
Servings: 2

Ingredients:

- Two cucumbers, chopped
- 1 tbsp. olive oil
- Salt and black pepper to the taste
- One red chili pepper, dried
- 1 tbsp. lemon juice
- 3 tbsp. walnuts, chopped
- 1 tbsp. balsamic vinegar
- 1 tsp. chives, chopped

Directions:

1. In a prepared bowl, mix the cucumbers with the oil and the rest of the ingredients, toss and serve as a side dish.

Nutrition:
Calories 121
Fat 2.3g
Fiber 2.0g
Carbs 6.7g
Protein 2.4 g

30. Cheesy Beet Salad

Preparation time: 10 minutes
Cooking time: 1 hour
Servings: 4

Ingredients:

- Four beets, peeled and cut into wedges
- 3 tbsp. olive oil
- Salt and black pepper to the taste
- ¼ cup lime juice
- Eight slices goat cheese, crumbled
- 1/3 cup walnuts, chopped
- 1 tbsp. chives, chopped

Directions:

1. In a roasting pan, combine the beets with the oil, salt, and pepper, toss and bake at 400 degrees F for 1 hour.
2. Cool the beets down, transfer them to a bowl, add the rest of the ingredients, toss and serve as a side salad.

Nutrition:
Calories: 156 Fat 4.2g
Fiber 3.4g Carbs 6.5g Protein 4 g

31. Rosemary Beets

Preparation time: 10 minutes
Cooking time: 20 minutes
Servings: 4

Ingredients:

- Four medium beets, peeled and cubed
- 1/3 cup balsamic vinegar
- 1 tsp. rosemary, chopped
- One garlic clove, minced
- ½ tsp. Italian seasoning
- 1 tbsp. olive oil

Directions:

1. Heat a pan put the oil over medium heat, add the beets and the rest of the ingredients, toss, and cook for 20 minutes.
2. Divide the mix between plates and serve as a side dish.

Nutrition:
Calories 165 Fat 3.4g
Fiber 4.5g
Carbs 11.3g
Protein 2.3g

32. Squash and Tomatoes Mix

Preparation time: 10 minutes
Cooking time: 20 minutes
Servings: 6

Ingredients:

- Five medium squash, cubed
- A pinch of salt and black pepper
- 3 tbsp. olive oil
- 1 cup pine nuts, toasted
- ¼ cup goat cheese, crumbled
- Six tomatoes, cubed
- ½ yellow onion, chopped
- 2 tbsp. cilantro, chopped
- 2 tbsp. lemon juice

Directions:

1. Heat a pan put the oil over medium heat, add the onion and pine nuts and cook for 3 minutes.
2. Add the squash and the rest of the ingredients, cook everything for 15 minutes, divide between plates and serve as a side dish.

Nutrition:
Calories 200
Fat 4.5g
Fiber 3.4g
Carbs 6.7g
Protein 4 g

33. Balsamic Eggplant Mix

Preparation time: 10 minutes
Cooking time: 20 minutes
Servings: 6

Ingredients:

- 1/3 cup chicken stock
- 2 tbsp. balsamic vinegar
- A pinch of salt and black pepper
- 1 tbsp. lime juice
- Two big eggplants, sliced
- 1 tbsp. rosemary, chopped
- ¼ cup cilantro, chopped
- 2 tbsp. olive oil

Directions:

1. In a roasting pan, combine the eggplants with the stock, the vinegar, and the rest of the ingredients, introduce the pan in the oven and bake at 390 degrees F for 20 minutes.
2. Divide the mix between plates and serve as a side dish.

Nutrition:
Calories 201
Fat 4.5g
Fiber 3g
Carbs 5.4g
Protein 3 g

34. Sage Barley Mix

Preparation time: 10 minutes
Cooking time: 45 minutes
Servings: 4

Ingredients:

- 1 tbsp. olive oil
- One red onion, chopped
- 1 tbsp. leaves, chopped
- One garlic clove, minced
- 14 ounces barley
- ½ tbsp. parmesan, grated
- 6 cups veggie stock
- Salt and black pepper to the taste

Directions:

1. Heat a pan put the oil over medium heat, add the onion and garlic, stir and sauté for 5 minutes.
2. Add the sage, barley, and the rest of the ingredients except the parmesan, stir, bring to a simmer and cook for 40 minutes,
3. Add the parmesan, stir, and divide between plates.

Nutrition:
Calories 210,
Fat 6.5,
Fiber 3.4,
Carbs 8.6
Protein 3.4

35. Chickpeas and Beets Mix

Preparation time: 10 minutes
Cooking time: 25 minutes
Servings: 4

Ingredients:

- 3 tbsp. capers, drained and chopped
- Juice of 1 lemon
- Zest of 1 lemon, grated

- One red onion, chopped
- 3 tbsp. olive oil
- 14 ounces canned chickpeas, drained
- 8 ounces beets, peeled and cubed
- 1 tbsp. parsley, chopped
- Salt and pepper to the taste

Directions:

1. Heat a pan put the oil over medium heat, add the onion, lemon zest, lemon juice, and the capers and sauté for 5 minutes.
2. Add the rest of the ingredients then stir and cook over medium-low heat for 20 minutes more.
3. Divide the mix between plates and serve as a side dish.

Nutrition:
Calories 199 Fat 4.5g
Fiber 2.3g Carbs 6.5g Protein 3.3 g

36. Pesto Broccoli Quinoa

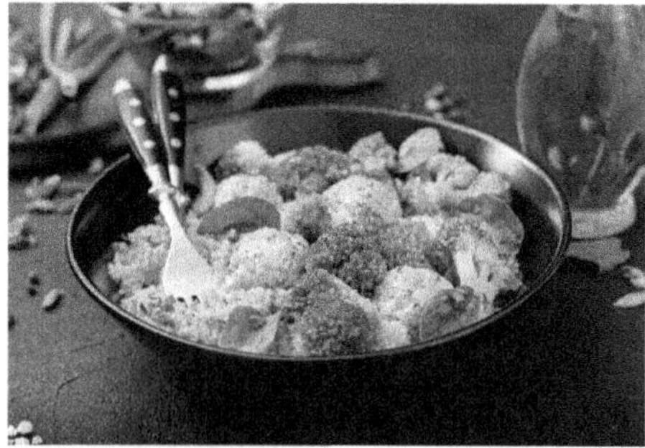

Preparation time: 10 minutes
Cooking time: 30 minutes
Servings: 4

Ingredients:

- Two and ½ cups quinoa
- Four and ½ cups veggie stock
- A pinch of salt and black pepper
- 2 tbsp. basil pesto
- 2 cups mozzarella cheese, shredded
- 1 pound broccoli florets
- 1/3 cup parmesan, grated
- Two green onions, chopped

Directions:

1. In a baking pan, combine the quinoa with the stock and the rest of the ingredients except the parmesan and the mozzarella and toss.
2. Sprinkle the cheese on top and bake everything at 400 degrees F and bake for 30 minutes.
3. Divide between plates and serve as a side dish.

Nutrition:
Calories 181 Fat 3.4g
Fiber 3.2g Carbs 8.6g
Protein 7.6 g

CHAPTER 5:

Seafood

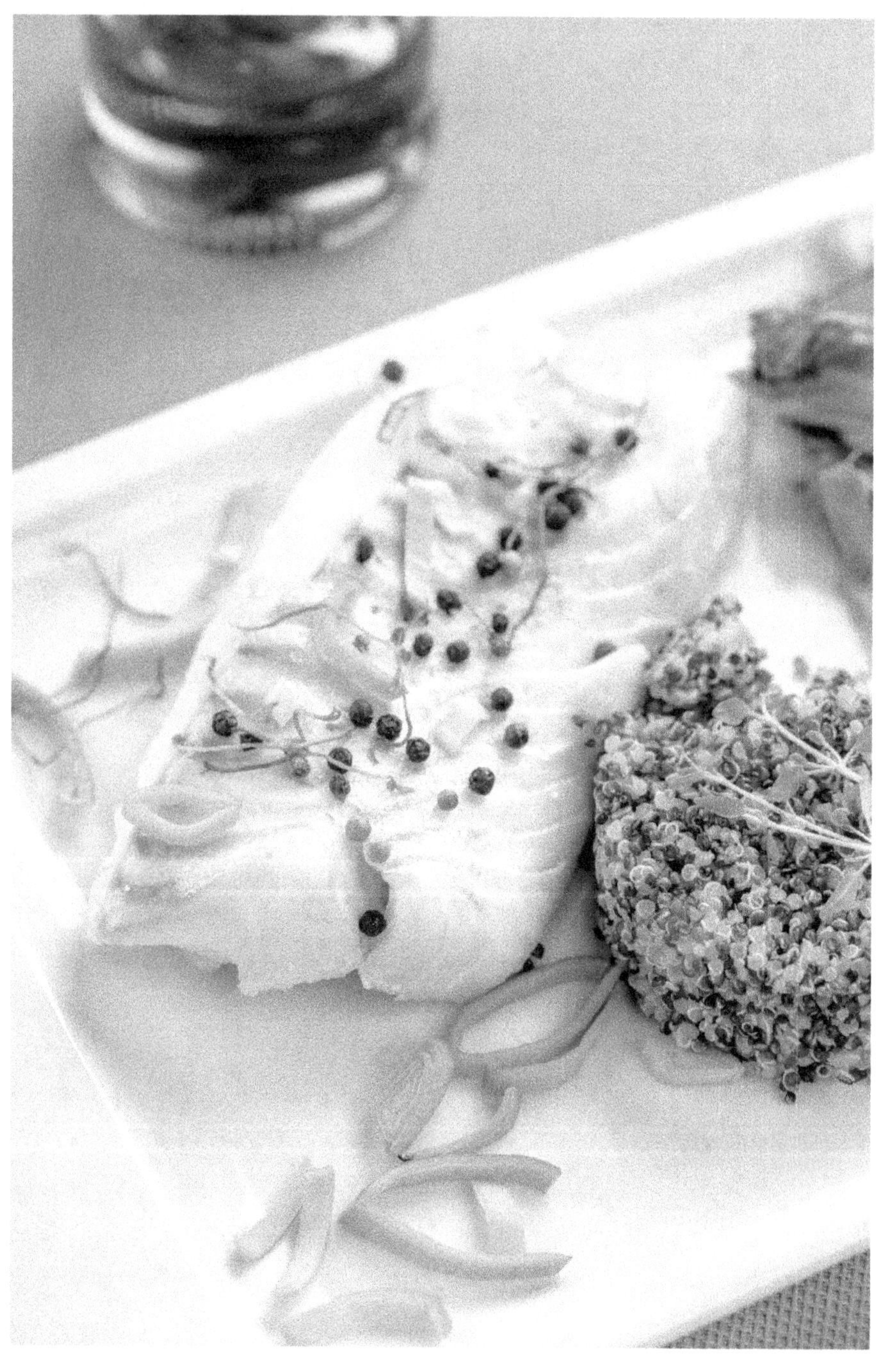

1.   Fish and Orzo

Preparation time: 10 minutes
Cooking time: 35 minutes
Servings: 4

Ingredients:

- 1 tsp. garlic, minced
- 1 tsp. red pepper, crushed
- Two shallots, chopped
- 1 tbsp. olive oil
- 1 tsp. anchovy paste
- 1 tbsp. oregano, chopped
- 2 tbsp. black olives, pitted and chopped
- 2 tbsp. capers, drained
- 15 ounces canned tomatoes, crushed
- A pinch of salt and black pepper
- Four cod fillets, boneless
- 1-ounce feta cheese, crumbled
- 1 tbsp. parsley, chopped
- 3 cups chicken stock
- 1 cup orzo pasta
- Zest of 1 lemon, grated

Directions:

1. Heat a pan put the oil over medium heat; add the garlic, red pepper, and the shallots and sauté for 5 minutes.
2. Add the anchovy paste, oregano, black olives, capers, tomatoes, salt, and pepper, stir and cook for 5 minutes more.
3. Add the cod fillets, sprinkle the cheese and the parsley on top, introduce in the oven and bake at 375 degrees F for 15 minutes more.
4. Meanwhile, put the stock in a pot, bring to a boil over medium heat, add the orzo and the lemon zest, bring to a simmer, cook for 10 minutes, fluff with a fork, and divide between plates.
5. Top each serving with the fish mix and serve.

Nutrition:
Calories 402
Fat 21g
Fiber 8g
Carbs 21g
Protein 31g

2.   Baked Sea Bass

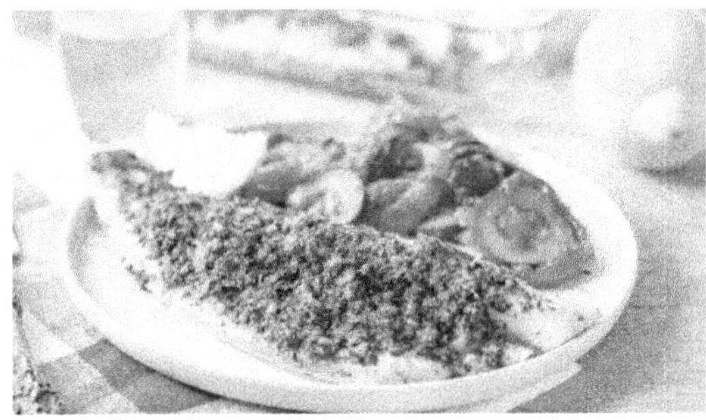

Preparation time: 10 minutes
Cooking time: 12 minutes
Servings: 4

Ingredients:

- Four sea bass fillets, boneless
- Salt and black pepper to the taste
- 2 cups potato chips, crushed
- 1 tbsp. mayonnaise

Directions:

1. Put seasonings on the fish fillets with salt and pepper, brush with the mayonnaise, and dredge each in the potato chips.
2. Arrange the fillets on a baking sheet lined with parchment paper and bake at 400 degrees F for 12 minutes.
3. Divide the fish between plates and serve with a side salad.

Nutrition
Calories: 228
Fat: 8.6g
Fiber: 0.6g
Carbs: 9.3g
Protein: 25g

3.   Fish and Tomato Sauce

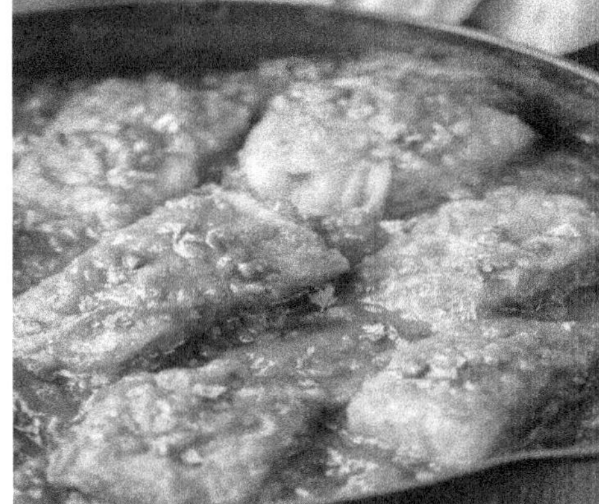

Preparation time: 10 minutes

Cooking time: 30 minutes
Servings: 4

Ingredients:

- Four cod fillets, boneless
- Two garlic cloves, minced
- 2 cups cherry tomatoes, halved
- 1 cup chicken stock
- A pinch of salt and black pepper
- ¼ cup basil, chopped

Directions:

1. Put the tomatoes, garlic, salt, and pepper in a pan, heat up over medium heat, and cook for 5 minutes.
2. Add the fish and the rest of the ingredients, bring to a simmer, cover the pan and cook for 25 minutes.
3. Divide the mix between plates and serve.

Nutrition
Calories 180
Fat 1.9g
Fiber 1.4g
Carbs 5.3g
Protein 33.8g

4.   Halibut and Quinoa Mix

Preparation time: 10 minutes
Cooking time: 12 minutes
Servings: 4

Ingredients:

- Four halibut fillets, boneless
- 2 tbsp. olive oil
- 1 tsp. Rosemary, dried
- 2 tsp. cumin, ground
- 1 tbsp. coriander, ground
- 2 tsp. cinnamon powder
- 2 tsp. oregano, dried
- A pinch of salt and black pepper
- 2 cups quinoa, cooked
- 1 cup cherry tomatoes, halved
- One avocado, peeled, pitted, and sliced
- One cucumber, cubed
- ½ cup black olives, pitted and sliced
- Juice of 1 lemon

Directions:

1. In a bowl, combine the fish with rosemary, cumin, coriander, cinnamon, oregano, salt, pepper, and toss.
2. Heat a pan put the oil over medium heat, add the fish, and sear for 2 minutes on each side.
3. Introduce the pan in the oven and bake the fish at 425 degrees F for 7 minutes.
4. Meanwhile, in a bowl, mix the quinoa with the remaining ingredients, toss and divide between plates.
5. Add the fish next to the quinoa mix and serve right away.

Nutrition
Calories 364
Fat 15.4g
Fiber 11.2g
Carbs 56.4g
Protein 24.5g

5.   Lemon and Dates Barramundi

Preparation time: 10 minutes
Cooking time: 12 minutes
Servings: 2

Ingredients:

- Two barramundi fillets, boneless
- One shallot, sliced
- Four lemon slices
- Juice of ½ lemon
- Zest of 1 lemon, grated
- 2 tbsp. olive oil
- 6 ounces baby spinach
- ¼ cup almonds, chopped
- Four dates, pitted and chopped
- ¼ cup parsley, chopped
- Salt and black pepper to the taste

Directions:

1. Put seasoning to the fish with salt and pepper and arrange on two parchment paper pieces.
2. Top the fish with the lemon slices drizzle the lemon juice, and then top with the other ingredients except for the oil.
3. Drizzle 1 tbsp. oil over each fish mix, wrap the parchment paper around the

fish, shape it into packets and arrange them on a baking sheet.

4. Bake at temperature of 400 degrees F for about 12 minutes cool the mix a bit, unfold, divide everything between plates and serve.

Nutrition

Calories 232 Fat 16.5g

Fiber 11.1g Carbs 24.8g Protein 6.5g

6. Fish Cakes

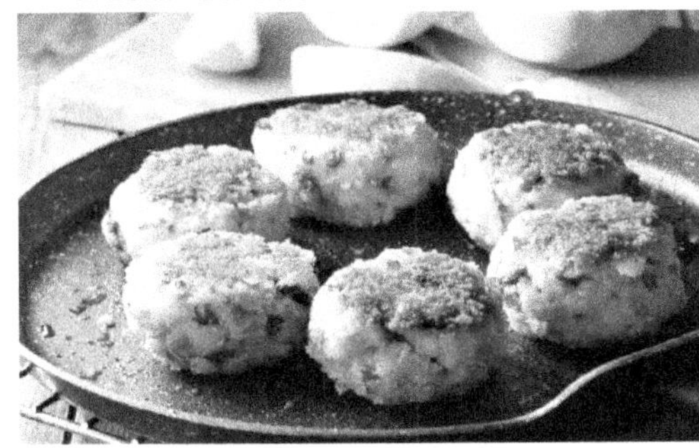

Preparation time: 10 minutes

Cooking time: 10 minutes

Servings: 6

Ingredients:

- 20 ounces canned sardines, drained and mashed well
- Two garlic cloves, minced
- 2 tbsp. dill, chopped
- One yellow onion, chopped
- 1 cup panko breadcrumbs
- One egg whisked
- A pinch of salt and black pepper
- 2 tbsp. lemon juice
- 5 tbsp. olive oil

Directions:

1. In a bowl, combine the sardines with the garlic, dill, and the rest of the ingredients except the oil, stir well and shape medium cakes out of this mix.
2. Heat a pan with the oil over medium-high heat, add the fish cakes, and cook for 5 minutes on each side.
3. Serve the cakes with a side salad.

Nutrition

Calories 288

Fat 12.8g

Fiber 10.2g

Carbs 22.2g

Protein 6.8g

7. Catfish Fillets and Rice

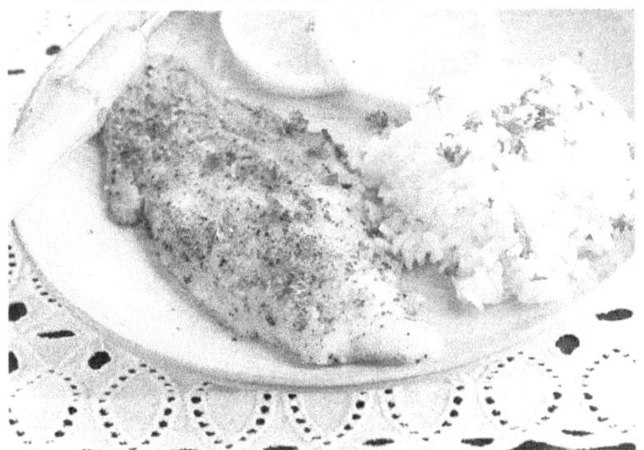

Preparation time: 10 minutes

Cooking time: 55 minutes

Servings: 2

Ingredients:

- Two catfish fillets, boneless
- 2 tbsp. Italian seasoning
- 2 tbsp. olive oil

For the rice:

- 1 cup brown rice
- 2 tbsp. olive oil
- One and ½ cups water
- ½ cup green bell pepper, chopped
- Two garlic cloves, minced
- ½ cup white onion, chopped
- 2 tsp. Cajun seasoning
- ½ tsp. garlic powder
- Salt and black pepper to the taste

Directions:

1. Heat a pot with 2 tbsp. oil over medium heat then add the onion, garlic, garlic powder, salt, and pepper and sauté for 5 minutes.
2. Add the rice, water, bell pepper, and seasoning to a simmer and cook over medium heat for 40 minutes.
3. Heat a pan with 2 tbsp. oil over medium heat, add the fish and the Italian seasoning and cook for 5 minutes on each side.
4. Divide the rice between plates, add the fish on top and serve.

Nutrition

Calories 261 Fat 17.6g
Fiber 12.2g Carbs 24.8g Protein 12.5g

8.   Halibut Pan

Preparation time: 10 minutes
Cooking time: 20 minutes
Servings: 4

Ingredients:

- Four halibut fillets, boneless
- One red bell pepper, chopped
- 2 tbsp. olive oil
- One yellow onion, chopped
- Four garlic cloves, minced
- ½ cup chicken stock
- 1 tsp. basil, dried
- ½ cup cherry tomatoes halved
- 1/3 cup of kalamata olives, pitted and halved
- Salt and black pepper to the taste

Directions:

1. Heat a pan put the oil over medium heat, add the fish, cook for 5 minutes on each side, and divide between plates.
2. Add the onion, bell pepper, garlic, and tomatoes to the pan, stir and sauté for 3 minutes.
3. Add salt, pepper, and the rest of the ingredients, toss, cook for 3 minutes more, divide next to the fish and serve.

Nutrition
Calories 253
Fat 8g
Fiber 1g
Carbs 5g
Protein 28g

Ingredients:

- ½ cup pecans, chopped
- 2 cups baby arugula
- 1 cup corn
- ¼ pound smoked salmon, skinless, boneless, and cut into small chunks
- 2 tbsp. olive oil
- 2 tbsp. lemon juice
- Sea salt and black pepper to the taste

Directions:

1. In a salad bowl, combine the salmon with the corn and the rest of the ingredients, toss, and serve right away.

Nutrition
Calories 284 Fat 18.4g
Fiber 5.4g
Carbs 22.6g
Protein 17.4g

9.   Cod and Mushrooms Mix

Preparation time: 10 minutes
Cooking time: 25 minutes
Servings: 4

Ingredients:

- Two cod fillets, boneless
- 4 tbsp. olive oil
- 4 ounces mushrooms, sliced
- Sea salt and black pepper to the taste
- 12 cherry tomatoes, halved
- 8 ounces lettuce leaves, torn
- One avocado, pitted, peeled, and cubed
- One red chili pepper, chopped
- 1 tbsp. cilantro, chopped
- 2 tbsp. balsamic vinegar
- 1-ounce feta cheese, crumbled

Directions:

1. Put the fish in a roasting pan, brush it with 2 tbsp. oil, sprinkle with the salt and pepper all over, and broil under medium-high heat for 15 minutes. Meanwhile, heat a pan with the rest of the oil over medium heat, add the mushrooms, stir and sauté for 5 minutes.
2. Add the rest of the ingredients, toss, cook for 5 minutes more, and divide between plates.
3. Top with the fish and serve right away.

Nutrition
Calories 257
Fat 10g
Fiber 3.1g
Carbs 24.3g
Protein 19.4 g

10.   Sesame Shrimp Mix

Preparation time: 10 minutes
Cooking time: 0 minutes
Servings: 4

Ingredients:

- 2 tbsp. lime juice
- 3 tbsp. teriyaki sauce
- 2 tbsp. olive oil
- 8 cups baby spinach
- 14 ounces shrimp, cooked, peeled, and deveined
- 1 cup cucumber, sliced
- 1 cup radish, sliced
- ¼ cup cilantro, chopped
- 2 tsp. sesame seeds, toasted

Directions:

1. In a prepared bowl, mix the shrimp with the lime juice, spinach, and the rest of the ingredients, toss and serve cold.

Nutrition
Calories 177
Fat 9g
Fiber 7.1g
Carbs 14.3g
Protein 9.4g

11.   Olive Oil Poached Cod

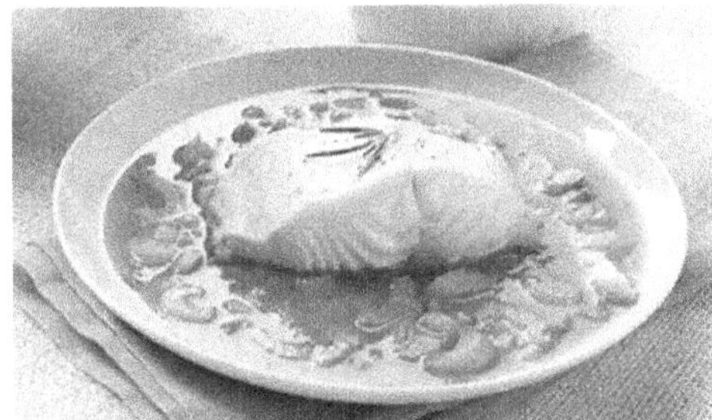

Preparation time: 5 minutes.
Cooking time: 10 minutes.
Servings: 4.

Ingredients:

- 2 tsp. of Lemon Juice.
- 4 Of 6 Oz of Cod Fillets.
- 3 Cups of Olive Oil.
- 1 tsp. of Lemon Zest.
- 1 tbsp. of Salt.

Directions:

1. Wash the fillets and put them on a paper towel.
2. Put oil inside a big pot, add the fish fillets to poach for about 6 minutes, or the fish color changes to opaque.
3. Take the fish out of the oil and add salt to it. Put some of the left-over warm oil on the fish, add lemon juice with it. Add zest by sprinkling. It is ready to be served.

Nutrition:
Calories: 305
Carbs: 10g
Fat: 15g
Protein: 31g

12.   Pistachio-Crusted Halibut

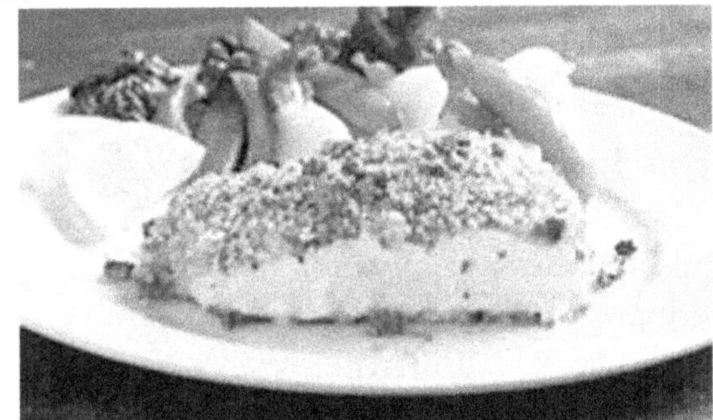

Preparation Time: 15 minutes
Cooking Time: 20 minutes
Servings: 4

Ingredients:

- 4 (6-Oz) Halibut Fillets with Skin Removed.
- ½ Cup Shelled Unsalted Pistachios (Chopped).
- 4 tsp. Fresh Parsley (Chopped).
- 1 Cup Bread Crumbs.
- ¼ Cup Extra-Virgin Olive Oil.
- 2 tsp. Grated Orange Zest.
- 1 Tsp. Grated Lime Zest.
- ½ Tsp. Pepper.
- 4 tsp. of Dijon Mustard.
- 11/2 of Salt.

Directions:

1. Preheat the oven to 4000F.

2. In the food processor, add pistachio, zest, bread crumbs, parsley, and oil. Pulse until the ingredients are well combined.
3. Rinse the fish and pat dry with a paper towel. Season the fillet with salt and pepper.
4. Brush the fish with mustard and divide the pistachio mix evenly with some on top of the fish. Press down the mixture to allow the crust to adhere.
5. Lining the baking sheet with crusted paper, arrange the crusted fish, and bake for 20minutes or until the fillet is golden brown. Leave for 5 minutes to cool, and then serve.

Nutrition:
Calories: 231
Carbs: 31.5g
Protein: 5.8g
Fat: 9.50g

13. Red Mullet Savaro Style

Preparation Time: 20 minutes
Cooking Time: 15 minutes
Servings: 4

Ingredients:

- 4(1/2-Pound) Red Mullet (Cleaned, Scaled, And Gutted).
- 2 Tsp. of Salt.
- 2/3 Cup of Olive Oil.
- 2 Tbsps. Of Rosemary.
- 8 Cloves of Finely Diced Garlic.
- 2/3 Cup of Red Wine Vinegar.

Directions:

1. Massage the fish with salt and leave for 20minutes.
2. Mix with flour and set aside. Add 1/3 cup of oil to the frying pan and heat over medium-high heat until it is hot; fry each fish 4-5 minutes per side. Set aside.
3. Pour the rest of the oil into another frying pan and add rosemary; fry until it turns an olive color, then remove from the oil.
4. Add garlic to the oil and stir until it turns golden. Add the vinegar and stir until the

sauce thickens and is bittersweet. Pour the source over the fish and serve.

Nutrition:
Calories: 150 Carbs: 2.1g
Fat: 8g Protein: 25g

14. Spinach-Stuffed Sole

Preparation Time: 5 minutes
Cooking Time: 20 minutes
Servings: 4

Ingredients:

- 4 (6-Oz) Of Sole Fillets.
- 4 Scallions with Ends Trimmed and Sliced.
- A 1-Pound Package of Frozen Spinach (Thawed).
- 1 tsp. of Salt.
- 3tsps. of Chopped Fennel.
- ½ tsp. Pepper.
- 1tsp Sweet Paprika.
- 2 Tbsps. Of Lemon.

Directions:

1. Preheat the oven to 4000F.
2. Put a small pan set on medium heat, and then add 2 tbsp. of oil and heat for 3osonds.
3. Add the scallion and cook for 3-4 minutes; allow it to cool.
4. In a bowl, add scallion, spinach, pepper, ½ tsp. of salt, and ¼ tsp. of pepper. Mix the ingredients.
5. Rinse and dry the fillet using a paper towel. Massage the fish with oil and sprinkle with pepper, paprika, and 2 tbsp. of lemon.
6. Spread the spinach fillings on the fillets, roll up each fillet starting from the wide-angle and secure each fillet with toothpicks.
7. Bake for 15-20 minutes. Remove the toothpick and sprinkle with lemon zest. Serve immediately.

Nutrition:
Calories: 174
Carb: 1g
Fat: 6g

Protein: 39g

15. Grilled Sardines

Preparation Time: 5 minutes
Cooking Time: 15 minutes
Servings: 4

Ingredients:

- 3 Tbsps. Of Vegetable Oil.
- ¾ Tsp. Of Pepper.
- 11/2 Tsp. Of Dried Oregano.
- 3 Tbsps. Of Lemon Juice.
- ½ Cup of Extra-Virgin Olive Oil (Divided).
- 2 Tsp. Of Salt.
- Clean Gutted and Scaled 2 Pounds of Fresh Sardine (the Head Removed)

Directions:

1. Preheat your set to a medium-high heat.
2. Rinse the sardine and pat it dry with a paper towel, then brush with olive oil on both sides. Sprinkle with pepper and salt on both sides.
3. Wipe the grill surface with oil. Place each sardine on the grill and grill for 2-3 minutes; while grilling, drizzle the sardine with olive oil and lemon juice.
4. Sprinkle with oregano and serve.

Nutrition:
Calories: 231
Carb: 0.6g
Protein: 26g
Fat: 13.6g

16. Halibut Roulade

Preparation Time: 5 minutes
Cooking Time: 10 minutes
Servings: 6

Ingredients:

- 1lbs of Halibut Fillet.
- ½ Pound Shrimp.
- 3 Limes.
- ½ Bunch Cilantro.
- 3 Cloves Garlic.
- ½ Leeks.
- 1 tbsp. Of Olive Oil.
- Freshly-Cracked Black Pepper.
- 1 Cup of Seafood Demi-Glace Reduction Sauce.

Directions:

1. Before starting, soak 12 wooden skewers in water for a minimum of 2 hours. Preheat the grill.
2. For the fillet, wash and chill, remove the shell and tail of the shrimp. Slice the shrimp in half along the length and remove the vein.
3. Squeeze two limes for juice and cut one into wedges. Grate the rind for zest.
4. Reserve some cilantro and chop the remaining ones. Slice the leek and mince the garlic.
5. Cut the halibut fillet across the length to about ½-3/4 inch thick. Spread and layer with shrimp, zest, cilantro, leek, and garlic, and carefully roll-up.
6. Cut the fillet into six pinwheels and insert two skewers into each pinwheel, forming X. brush with oil and grill for 4minutes per side or until it is golden brown.
7. Drizzle with oil and garnish with the remaining cilantro, zest, ½ tsp. of pepper. Serve with demi-glace reduction sauce.

Nutrition:
Calories: 342 Carb: 11g Protein: 46g

17. Glazed Broiled Salmon

Preparation Time: 20 minutes
Cooking Time: 20 minutes
Servings: 4-6
Ingredients:
Glaze:

- 2 Tbsp. Dark Brown Sugar.
- 4 Tsp. Dijon Mustard.
- 1 Tbsp. Soy Sauce.
- 1 Tsp. Rice Vinegar.

Salmon:

- 2 Medium Size Salmon Fillets.

Directions:

1. Preheat oven to broil.

2. Mix glaze ingredients.
3. Clean and de-bone salmon.
4. Coat with glaze the side of the salmon. Place on a baking sheet.
5. Broil salmon within 8-10 inches of the coils, be careful not to get too close; you don't want it cooking too fast.
6. It is done when it opaque and flakes easily in the center.

Nutrition:
Calories: 10 Carb: 0.86g
Protein: 0.31g Fat: 0.59g

18. Honey-Mustard Roasted Salmon

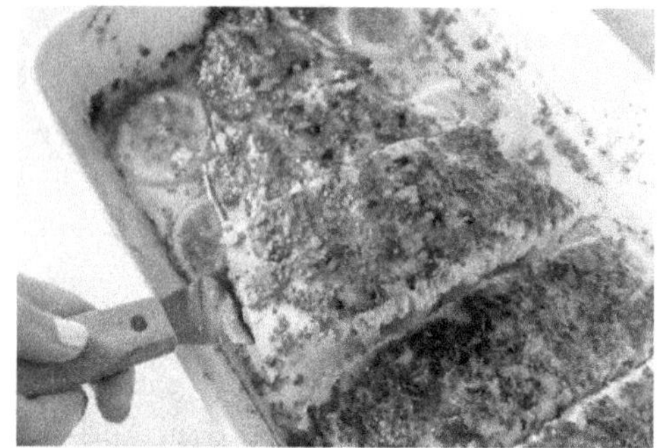

Preparation Time: 5 minutes
Cooking Time: 25 minutes
Servings: 6

Ingredients:

- Cooking Spray.
- 1 Lemon Sliced.
- 1 (3-Lb.) Salmon Fillet.
- Kosher Salt.
- Freshly Ground Black Pepper.
- 1/2 C. Whole Grain Mustard.
- 1/4 C. Extra-Virgin Olive Oil.
- 1/4 C. Honey.
- 2 Cloves Garlic, Minced.
- 1/2 Tsp. Red Pepper Flakes.

Directions:

1. Freshly chopped parsley for serving.
2. Preheat oven set to 400° and grease a 9"-x-13" baking dish with cooking spray. Place lemon slices on the bottom of the dish and place salmon on top. Put seasoning with salt and pepper.
3. In a medium bowl, whisk together mustard, oil, honey, garlic, and red pepper flakes. Put seasonings with salt and pepper, then pour the sauce over salmon.
4. Roast salmon until cooked through and flakes easily with a fork, 20 minutes.
5. Turn oven to broil and broil another 5 minutes, if desired.
6. Garnish with parsley before serving.

Nutrition:
Calories: 115 Carb: 19.74g
Protein: 1.49g   Fat: 4.14g

19. Asian-Inspired Tuna Lettuce Wraps

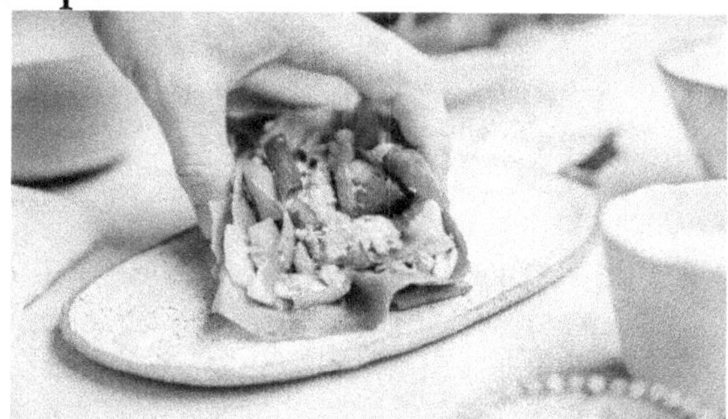

Preparation Time: 30 minutes
Cooking Time: 0 minutes
Servings: 6-7

Ingredients:

For the wraps:

- 1 Head Butter Lettuce or Romaine Lettuce
- 3 Packets Good Catch Foods Tuna
- 1 Large Carrot, Peeled into Ribbons
- 1 Large Red Pepper, Sliced
- 1/4 cup Green Onions, Roughly Chopped
- A Handful of Fresh Cilantro

For the sauce:

- 1 Tbsp. Fresh Ginger, Grated
- 2 Cloves of Garlic, Grated
- 1 1/2 Tbsp. Soy Sauce or Coconut Aminos
- 2 Tbsp. Sesame Oil and Seeds
- Juice of Half A Lime
- 1 Tbsp. Rice Wine Vinegar
- 2 Tbsp. Vegetable Oil

- 2 Tbsp. Maple Syrup

Directions:

1. To a prepared medium-sized bowl, add your Good Catch Foods Tuna and all your sauce ingredients. Mash up the stir gently using a fork and mix it well. Set aside to marry for 15 minutes until your lettuce wraps are assembled.
2. While you wait, prepare all your choice of vegetables and set them aside.
3. If you like to add 2-3 pieces of butter lettuce or one piece of Romaine as the base to create your lettuce wraps, then begin filling with veggies + tuna!
4. Enjoy like you would at taco (butter lettuce) or pizza (romaine lettuce).

Nutrition:
Calories: 81
Carb: 7.52g
Protein: 1.18g
Fat: 5.42g

20. Mediterranean Grilled Sea Bass

Preparation Time: 10 minutes
Cooking Time: 12 minutes
Servings: 4

Ingredients:

- Two lemons
- 3 tbsp. olive oil
- 1 tbsp. chopped fresh oregano leaves
- 1 tsp. ground coriander
- 1 1/4 tsp. salt
- Two whole sea bass, cleaned and scaled (about 1 1/2 lbs. each)
- 1/4 tsp. ground black pepper
- Two large oregano sprigs

Directions:

1. Preheat gas grill over medium heat.
2. For the meantime, from 1 lemon, grate 1 tbsp. peel and squeeze 2 tbsp. juice. Cut half of the remaining lemon into slices, the other half into wedges. In a small bowl, stir lemon juice and peel, oil, chopped oregano, coriander, and 1/4 tsp. salt.

3. Rinse fish and pat dry use paper towels. Make three slashes on both sides of each fish. Sprinkle inside and out with pepper and the remaining 1 tsp. salt. Put lemon slices and oregano sprigs inside fish cavities. Place fish in a 13" by 9" glass baking dish. Rub half of the oil mixture over the fish's outsides; reserve the remaining oil mixture for drizzling overcooked fish. Let rest at room temperature for 15 minutes.
4. Lightly grease grill rack; place fish on hot rack. Cover grill and cook fish for 12 to 14 minutes or until fish just turns opaque throughout and thickest part flakes easily when tested with a fork, turning fish over once.
5. To serve, place fish on the cutting board. Working with one fish at a time, with a knife, cut along backbone from head to tail. Slide wide metal spatula or cake server under the top fillet's front section and lift off from backbone; transfer to a platter. Gently pull-out backbone and rib bones from bottom fillet and discard. Transfer bottom fillet to platter. Repeat with the second fish—drizzle fillets with the remaining oil mixture. Serve with lemon wedges.

Nutrition:
Calories305
Protein: 40g
Carbohydrate: 1g
Fat: 15g
Fiber: 0g

21. Peppercorn-Seared Tuna Steaks

Preparation Time: 15 minutes
Cooking Time: 10 minutes
Servings: 4

Ingredients:

- 1 Tbsp. Sesame Seed Oil or More, As Needed
- 1 Tsp. Olive Oil Plus More, If Needed
- 4 8 oz. of Tuna Steaks Fresh, 8 To 12 Oz.

- ¼ Cup Black Peppercorns Crushed, Or Black Sesame Seeds
- ¼ Cup Sesame Seeds White
- 4 Cups Baby Spinach Fresh, Rinsed, And Dried
- ½ Cup Pine Nuts Toasted
- ½ Cup Goat Cheese Crumbled
- ½ Cup Strawberry Vinaigrette or More, If Desired
- ½ Cup Pea Sprouts or Bean Sprouts

Directions:
1. Make the strawberry vinaigrette.
2. Pat the tuna steaks dry use a paper towel.
3. Rub the tuna on all sides with sesame oil.
4. On a large platter, combine the crushed peppercorns and sesame seeds. When completely coated, dredge the tuna steaks in the pepper/sesame mixture.
5. In a non-stick skillet set over a medium-high flame, heat the olive oil.
6. Put the encrusted tuna steaks into the hot skillet and cook for 11/2 minutes, working in batches of two at a time. Turn around, and cook the other side for another 1½ minutes. Cook 2 minutes per side for medium-rare ones.
7. Remove from heat, and if cool enough to handle, cut into 1/2-inch-thick slices against the grain.
8. For the meantime, in a prepared large salad bowl, put the spinach and top with the toasted pine nuts and goat cheese. Toss with about ¾ cup of the vinaigrette.
9. For serving bowls, split the dressed spinach. Add the sliced tuna, circularly, on top of the salad.
10. Drizzle some more of the vinaigrette over the top of the tuna and add to the middle of the salad a small bunch of pea sprouts. Serve at once.

Nutrition:
Calories: 290kcal Carbohydrates: 6g
Protein: 10g Fat: 4g Cholesterol: 13mg

22. Crispy Tilapia with Mango Salsa

Preparation Time: 15 minutes

Cooking Time: 10 minutes
Servings: 4

Ingredients:
Mango salsa:
- 1 Medium (1 Cup) Mango, Coarsely Chopped
- 2 Tbsp. Finely Chopped Red Bell Pepper
- 1 Tbsp. Finely Chopped Red Onion
- 2 Tsp. Finely Chopped Seeded Jalapeño Chile Pepper
- 1 Tsp. Finely Chopped Fresh Cilantro

Fish:
- 1 to 1 1/2 pounds fresh or frozen tilapia fillets, thawed if frozen
- 1 cup panko bread crumbs
- 2 tsp. chopped fresh parsley
- 1/2 tsp. salt
- 1/4 cup milk
- One large land o lake® egg
- 1/4 cup land o lakes® butter

Directions:
1. Combine all salsa ingredients in a bowl. Cover; refrigerate for at least 1 hour.
2. Rinse fish fillets; pat dry use paper towels.
3. Mix parsley, bread crumbs, and salt in a 9-inch pie pan. Whisk together milk and egg in another 9-inch pie pan. Dip fillets in egg mixture; then into bread crumb mixture, turning to coat thoroughly.
4. Melt butter in a 12-inch skillet until sizzling; add coated fish fillets. Cook over medium heat, turning once, 8-10 minutes or until fish flakes with a fork. Serve with salsa.

Nutrition:
Calories: 430kcal Carbohydrates: 46g
Protein: 26.63g Fat: 15.58g
Cholesterol: 57mg

23. Air-Fried Flounder Fillets

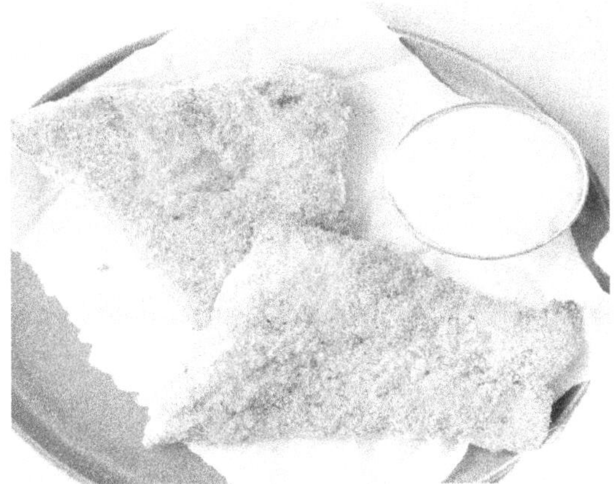

Preparation Time: 5 minutes
Cooking Time: 12 minutes
Serving: 4

Ingredients

- 2 cups unsweetened almond milk
- ½ tsp. onion powder
- ½ tsp. garlic powder
- 4 (4-ounce / 113-g) flounder fillets
- ½ cup chickpea flour
- ½ cup plain yellow cornmeal
- ¼ tsp. cayenne pepper
- Freshly ground black pepper, to taste

Directions

1. Whisk together the almond milk, onion powder, and garlic powder in a large bowl until smooth.
2. Add the flounder, coating well on both sides, and let marinate for about 20 minutes.
3. Meanwhile, combine the chickpea flour, cornmeal, cayenne, and pepper in a shallow dish.
4. Dredge each piece of flounder fillets in the flour mixture until completely coated.
5. Preheat the air fryer set to 380°F (193°C).
6. Arrange the coated flounder fillets in the basket and cook for 12 minutes, flipping them halfway through.
7. Remove from the basket and serve on a plate.

Tip: If an air fryer isn't available, you can place the flounder fillets on a rimmed baking sheet and broil for 12 minutes, flipping once halfway through.

Nutrition

Calories: 228 Fat: 5.7g
Protein: 28.2g Carbs: 15.5g
Fiber: 2.0g Sodium: 240mg

24.   Minute Cod with Parsley Pistou

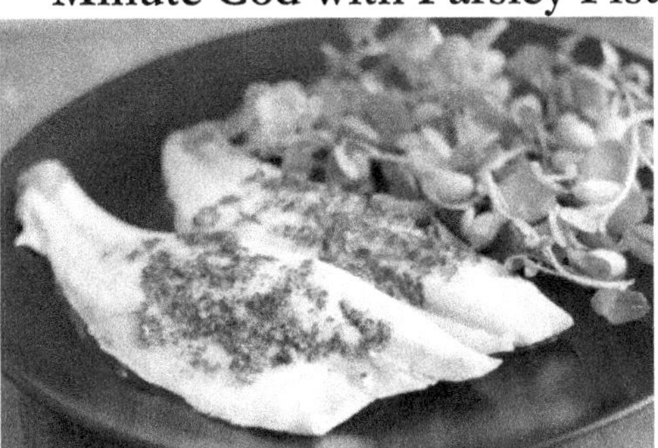

Preparation Time: 15 minutes
Cooking Time: 10 minutes
Serving: 4

Ingredients

- 1 cup packed roughly and chopped fresh flat-leaf Italian parsley
- Zest and juice of 1 lemon
- 1 to 2 small garlic cloves, minced
- 1 tsp. salt
- ½ tsp. freshly ground black pepper
- 1 cup extra-virgin olive oil, divided
- 1 pound (454 g) cod fillets, cut into four equal-sized pieces

Directions

1. Make the pistou: Place the parsley, lemon zest and juice, garlic, salt, and pepper in a food processor until finely chopped.
2. With the running food processor, slowly drizzle a ¾ cup of olive oil until a thick sauce form. Set aside.
3. Heat the remaining ¼ cup of olive oil in a large skillet over medium-high heat.
4. Add the cod fillets, cover, and cook each side for 4 to 5 minutes, until browned and cooked through.
5. Remove the cod fillets from the heat to a plate and top each with generous spoonful of the prepared pistou. Serve immediately.

Tip: You can serve the pistou on steamed vegetables, toasted whole-wheat bread, salads, and other grilled meats or seafood.

Nutrition
Calories: 580
Fat: 54.6g
Protein: 21.1g
Carbs: 2.8g
Fiber: 1.0g

25.   Simple Fried Cod Fillets
Preparation Time: 5 minutes
Cooking Time: 10 minutes
Serving: 4

Ingredients
- ½ cup all-purpose flour
- 1 tsp. garlic powder
- 1 tsp. salt
- 4 (4- to 5-ounce / 113- to 142-g) cod fillets
- 1 tbsp. extra-virgin olive oil

Directions
1. Mix together the flour, garlic powder, and salt in a shallow dish.
2. Put each piece of fish in the seasoned flour until they are evenly coated.
3. Heat the olive oil in a prepared medium skillet over medium-high heat.
4. Once hot, add the cod fillets and fry for 6 to 8 minutes, flipping the fish halfway through or until the fish is opaque and flakes easily.
5. Remove from the heat and serve on plates.

Tip: You can use various spices or herbs to season the flour, such as onion powder, paprika, black pepper, oregano, marjoram, or even tarragon.

Nutrition
Calories: 333
Fat: 18.8g
Protein: 21.2g
Carbs: 20.0g
Fiber: 5.7g

26.   Mediterranean Braised Cod with Vegetables
Preparation Time: 10 minutes
Cooking Time: 18 minutes
Serving: 2

Ingredients:
- 1 tbsp. olive oil
- ½ medium onion, minced
- Two garlic cloves, minced
- 1 tsp. oregano
- 1 (15-ounce / 425-g) can artichoke hearts in water, drained and halved
- 1 (15-ounce / 425-g) can diced tomatoes with basil
- ¼ cup pitted Greek olives, drained
- 10 ounces (284 g) wild cod
- Salt to taste
- Freshly ground black pepper, to taste

Directions:
1. In a skillet, heat the olive oil over medium-high heat.
2. Sauté the onion for about 5 minutes, stirring occasionally, or until tender.
3. Stir in the garlic and oregano and cook for 30 seconds more until fragrant.
4. Add the artichoke hearts, tomatoes, and olives and stir to combine. Top with the cod.
5. Cover and cook for 10 minutes, or until the fish flakes easily with a fork and juices run clear.
6. Sprinkle with salt and pepper. Serve warm.

Tip: The cod can be substituted with other lean white fish such as bass, tilapia, haddock, and halibut.

Nutrition:
Calories: 332
Fat: 10.5g
Protein: 29.2g
Carbs: 30.7g
Fiber: 8.0g

27.   Lemon-Parsley Swordfish

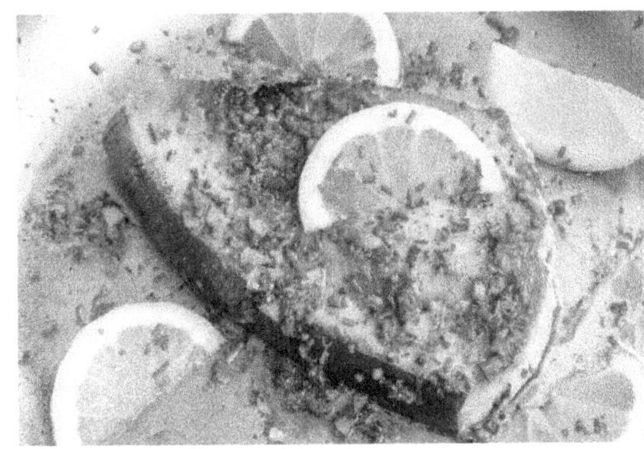

Preparation Time: 10 minutes
Cooking Time: 17 minutes
Serving: 4

Ingredients:

- 1 cup fresh Italian parsley
- ¼ cup lemon juice
- ¼ cup extra-virgin olive oil
- ¼ cup fresh thyme
- Two cloves garlic
- ½ tsp. salt
- Four swordfish steaks
- Olive oil spray

Directions:

1. Preheat the oven set to 450ºF (235ºC). Grease a large baking dish generously with olive oil spray.
2. Place the parsley, lemon juice, olive oil, thyme, garlic, and salt in a food processor and pulse until smoothly blended.
3. Arrange the swordfish steaks in the greased baking dish and spoon the parsley mixture over the top.
4. Bake in the preheated oven set to 17 to 20 minutes until flaky.
5. Divide the fish among four plates and serve hot.

Tips: If you prefer a milder flavor, you can substitute the fresh cilantro or basil for parsley.

Nutrition:
Calories: 396
Fat: 21.7g
Protein: 44.2g
Carbs: 2.9g
Fiber: 1.0g
Sodium: 494mg

28.   Baked Salmon with Tarragon Mustard Sauce

Preparation Time: 5 minutes
Cooking Time: 12 minutes
Serving: 4

Ingredients:

- 1¼ pounds (567 g) salmon fillet (skin on or removed), cut into four equal pieces
- ¼ cup Dijon mustard
- ¼ cup avocado oil mayonnaise
- Zest and juice of ½ lemon
- 2 tbsp. chopped fresh tarragon
- ½ tsp. salt
- ¼ tsp. freshly ground black pepper
- 4 tbsp. extra-virgin olive oil for serving

Directions:

1. Preheat the oven set to 425ºF (220ºC). Line a baking sheet with parchment paper.
2. Arrange the salmon pieces on the prepared baking sheet, skin-side down.
3. Stir together the mustard, avocado oil, mayonnaise, lemon zest and juice, tarragon, salt, and pepper in a small bowl. Spoon the mustard mixture over the salmon.
4. Bake at 10 to 12 minutes time, or until the top is golden and salmon is opaque in the center.
5. Divide the salmon among four plates and drizzle each top with 1 tbsp. of olive oil before serving.

Tip: You can use 1 to 2 tsp.—dried tarragon to replace the fresh tarragon.

Nutrition:
Calories: 386
Fat: 27.7g
Protein: 29.3g
Carbs: 3.8g
Fiber: 1.0g

29.   Baked Lemon Salmon

Preparation Time: 5 minutes
Cooking Time: 20 minutes
Serving: 4

Ingredients:

- ¼ tsp. dried thyme
- Zest and juice of ½ lemon
- ¼ tsp. salt
- ½ tsp. freshly ground black pepper
- 1 pound (454 g) salmon fillet
- Nonstick cooking spray

Directions:

1. Preheat the oven set to 425°F (220°C). Coat a baking sheet with nonstick cooking spray.
2. Mix the thyme, lemon zest and juice, salt, and pepper in a small bowl and stir to incorporate.
3. Arrange the salmon, skin-side down, on the coated baking sheet. Spoon the thyme mixture over the salmon and spread it all over.
4. Bake in the preheated oven set for approximately 15 to 20 minutes or until the fish flakes apart easily. Serve warm.
   Tip: To make this a complete meal, you can toss the cut-up asparagus, cauliflower, and broccoli with 1 tsp. olive oil in a large bowl until well coated and add them to the baking sheet.

Nutrition:
Calories: 162
Fat: 7.0g
Protein: 23.1g
Carbs: 1.0g

30. Baked Salmon with Basil and Tomato

Preparation Time: 10 minutes
Cooking Time: 20 minutes
Serving: 2

Ingredients:

- 2 (6-ounce / 170-g) boneless salmon fillets
- 1 tbsp. dried basil
- One tomato, thinly sliced
- 1 tbsp. olive oil
- 2 tbsp. grated Parmesan cheese
- Nonstick cooking spray

Directions:

1. Preheat the oven set at 375°F (190°C). Line a baking sheet with aluminum foil and mist with nonstick cooking spray.
2. Arrange the salmon fillets onto the aluminum foil and scatter with basil. Place the tomato slices on top and drizzle with olive oil. Top with the grated Parmesan cheese.
3. Bake for about 20 minutes time, or until the flesh is opaque and it flakes apart easily.
4. Remove from the oven and serve on a plate.

Nutrition:
Calories: 403
Fat: 26.5g
Protein: 36.3g
Carbs: 3.8g
Fiber: 0.1g

31. Salmon and Mushroom Hash with Pesto

Preparation Time: 15 minutes
Cooking Time: 20 minutes
Serving: 6

Ingredients:

Pesto:

- ¼ cup extra-virgin olive oil
- One bunch fresh basil
- Juice and zest of 1 lemon
- 1/3 cup water
- ¼ tsp. salt, plus additional as needed

Hash:

- 2 tbsp. extra-virgin olive oil
- 6 cups mixed mushrooms (brown, white, shiitake, cremini, portobello, etc.), sliced
- 1 pound (454 g) wild salmon, cubed

Directions:

1. Make the pesto: Pulse the olive oil, basil, juice and zest, water, and salt in a blender or food processor until smoothly blended. Set aside.

2. Heat the olive oil in a prepared large skillet over medium heat.

3. Stir-fry the mushrooms for 6 to 8 minutes, or until they begin to exude their juices.

4. Add the salmon and cook each side for 5 to 6 minutes until cooked through.

5. Fold in the prepared pesto and stir well. Taste and add additional salt as needed. Serve warm.

Tip: You can use coconut oil to replace the extra-virgin olive oil.

Nutrition:
Calories: 264
Fat: 14.7g
Protein: 7.0g
Carbs: 30.9g
Fiber: 4.0g

32. Spiced Citrus Sole

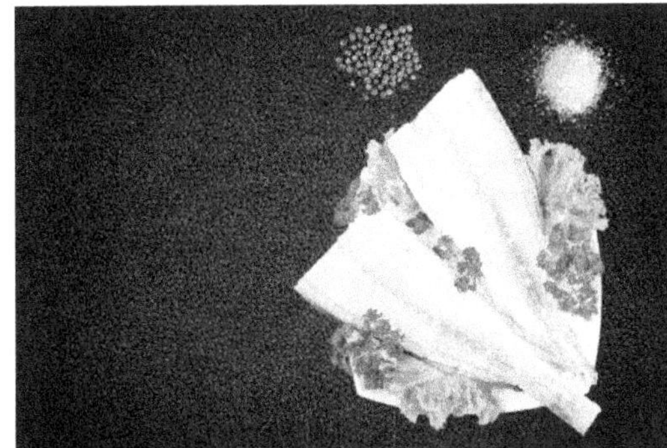

Preparation Time: 10 minutes
Cooking Time: 10 minutes
Serving: 4

Ingredients:

- 1 tsp. garlic powder
- 1 tsp. chili powder
- ½ tsp. lemon zest
- ½ tsp. lime zest
- ¼ tsp. smoked paprika
- ¼ tsp. freshly ground black pepper
- Pinch sea salt
- 4 (6-ounce / 170-g) sole fillets, patted dry
- 1 tbsp. extra-virgin olive oil
- 2 tsp. freshly squeezed lime juice

Directions:

1. Preheat the oven set at 450°F (235°C). Line a baking sheet with aluminum foil and set it aside.

2. Mix the garlic powder, chili powder, lemon zest, lime zest, paprika, pepper, and salt in a small bowl until well combined.

3. Arrange the sole fillets on the prepared baking sheet and rub the spice mixture all over the fillets until well coated. Drizzle over the filets with the olive oil and lime juice.

4. Bake in the preheated oven for about 8 minutes until flaky.

5. Remove from the heat to a plate and serve.

Tip: You can store the spice mixture in an airtight container for up to 2 weeks.

Nutrition:
Calories: 183 Fat: 5.0g Protein: 32.1g
Carbs: 0g

33. Braised Branzino with Wine Sauce

Preparation Time: 15 minutes
Cooking Time: 15 minutes
Serving: 2-3

Ingredients:

Sauce:

- ¾ cup dry white wine
- 2 tbsp. white wine vinegar
- 2 tbsp. cornstarch
- 1 tbsp. honey

Fish:

- One large branzino, butterflied and patted dry
- 2 tbsp. onion powder
- 2 tbsp. paprika
- ½ tbsp. salt
- 6 tbsp. extra-virgin olive oil, divided
- Four garlic cloves, thinly sliced
- Four scallions, both green and white parts, thinly sliced
- One large tomato, cut into ¼-inch cubes
- Four kalamata olives, pitted and chopped

Directions:

1. Make the sauce: Mix the white wine, vinegar, cornstarch, and honey in a bowl and keep stirring until the honey has dissolved. Set aside.
2. Make the fish: Place the fish on a clean work surface, skin-side down. Sprinkle the onion powder, paprika, and salt to season. Put 2 tbsp. of olive oil all over the fish.
3. Heat the pan put 2 tbsp. of olive oil in a large skillet over high heat until it shimmers.
4. Add the fish, skin-side up, to the skillet, and brown for about 2 minutes. Carefully flip the fish and cook for another 3 minutes. Remove from the heat to a plate and set aside.
5. Add the remaining 2 tbsp.—olive oil to the skillet and swirl to coat. Stir in the garlic cloves, scallions, tomato, and kalamata olives and sauté for 5 minutes. Pour in the prepared sauce and stir to combine.
6. Return the fish (skin-side down) to the skillet, flipping to coat in the sauce. Lower the heat to medium-low then cook for an additional 5 minutes until cooked through.
7. Using a slotted spoon, transfer the fish to a plate and serve warm.

Tip: If you have any leftovers, you can serve them with steamed brown rice or roasted potatoes.

Nutrition:
Calories: 1059
Fat: 71.9g
Protein: 46.2g
Carbs: 55.8g
Fiber: 5.1g

34. Baked Halibut Steaks with Vegetables

Preparation Time: 15 minutes
Cooking Time: 20 minutes
Serving: 4

Ingredients:

- 2 tsp. olive oil, divided
- One clove garlic, peeled and minced
- ½ cup minced onion
- 1 cup diced zucchini
- 2 cups diced fresh tomatoes
- 2 tbsp. chopped fresh basil
- ¼ tsp. salt
- ¼ tsp. ground black pepper
- 4 (6-ounce / 170-g) halibut steaks
- 1/3 cup crumbled feta cheese

Directions:

1. Preheat oven to 450°F (235°C). Coat a shallow baking dish lightly with 1 tsp. of olive oil.
2. In a medium saucepan, heat the remaining 1 tsp. of olive oil.
3. Add the garlic, onion, and zucchini and mix well. Cook for 5 minutes, stirring occasionally, or until the zucchini is softened.
4. Remove the saucepan from the heat and stir in the tomatoes, basil, salt, and pepper.
5. Place the halibut steaks in the coated baking dish in a single layer. Spread the zucchini mixture evenly over the steaks. Scatter the top with feta cheese.
6. Bake in the preheated oven for about 15 minutes, or until the fish flakes when pressed lightly with a fork. Serve hot.

Nutrition:
Calories: 258
Fat: 7.6g
Protein: 38.6g
Carbs: 6.5g
Fiber: 1.2g

35. Spicy Haddock Stew

Preparation Time: 15 minutes
Cooking Time: 35 minutes
Serving: 6

Ingredients:

- ¼ cup coconut oil
- 1 tbsp. minced garlic

- One onion, chopped
- Two celery stalks, chopped
- ½ fennel bulb, thinly sliced
- One carrot, diced
- One sweet potato, diced
- 1 (15-ounce / 425-g) can low-sodium diced tomatoes
- 1 cup coconut milk
- 1 cup low-sodium chicken broth
- ¼ tsp. red pepper flakes
- 12 ounces (340 g) haddock, cut into 1-inch chunks
- 2 tbsp. chopped fresh cilantro for garnish

Directions:

1. In a prepared large saucepan, heat the coconut oil over medium-high heat.
2. Add the garlic, onion, and celery and sauté for about 4 minutes, stirring occasionally, or until they are tender.
3. Stir in the fennel bulb, carrot, and sweet potato and sauté for 4 minutes more.
4. Add the diced tomatoes, coconut milk, chicken broth, and red pepper flakes and stir to incorporate, and then bring the mixture to a boil.
5. Once it starts to boil, turn the heat to low, bring to a simmer for about 15 minutes, or until the vegetables are fork-tender.
6. Add the haddock chunks and continue simmering for about 10 minutes or until the fish is cooked through.
7. Sprinkle the cilantro on top for garnish before serving.

Tip: If you prefer a bit of heat, you could add a bit of Chile.

Nutrition:
Calories: 276 Fat: 20.9g
Protein: 14.2g
Carbs: 6.8g

36. Cioppino (Seafood Tomato Stew)

Preparation Time: 10 minutes
Cooking Time: 20 minutes
Serving: 2

Ingredients:

- 2 tbsp. olive oil
- ½ small onion, diced
- ½ green pepper, diced
- 2 tsp. dried basil
- 2 tsp. dried oregano
- ½ cup dry white wine
- 1 (14.5-ounce / 411-g) can diced tomatoes with basil
- 1 (8-ounce / 227-g) can no-salt-added tomato sauce
- 1 (6.5-ounce / 184-g) can minced clams with their juice
- 8 ounces (227 g) peeled, deveined raw shrimp
- 4 ounces (113 g) any white fish (a thick piece works best)
- 3 tbsp. fresh parsley
- Salt to taste
- Freshly ground black pepper, to taste

Directions:

1. In a Dutch oven, heat the olive oil over medium heat.
2. Sauté the onion and green pepper for 5 minutes, or until tender.
3. Stir in the basil, oregano, wine, diced tomatoes, and tomato sauce and bring to a boil.
4. Once boiling, turn the heat to low and bring to a simmer for 5 minutes.
5. Add the clams, shrimp, and fish and cook for about 10 minutes, or until the shrimp are pink and cooked through.
6. Scatter with the parsley and add the salt and black pepper to taste.
7. Remove from the heat and serve warm.

Tip: You can prepare this stew's base in advance, but do not stir in the fish until just before serving.

Nutrition:
Calories: 221
Fat: 7.7g
Protein: 23.1g
Carbs: 10.9g
Fiber: 4.2g

37.　Lemon Grilled Shrimp

Preparation Time: 20 minutes
Cooking Time: 4-6 minutes
Serving: 4

Ingredients

- 2 tbsp. garlic, minced
- 3 tbsp. fresh Italian parsley, finely chopped
- ¼ cup extra-virgin olive oil
- ½ cup lemon juice
- 1 tsp. salt
- 2 pounds (907 g) jumbo shrimp (21 to 25), peeled and deveined

Special Equipment:

Four skewers, soaked in water for at least 30 minutes

Directions:

1. Whisk together the garlic, parsley, olive oil, lemon juice, and salt in a large bowl.
2. Add the shrimp to the bowl and toss well, making sure the shrimp are coated in the marinade. Set aside to sit for 15 minutes.
3. When ready, skewer the shrimps by piercing through the center. You can place about 5 to 6 shrimps on each skewer.
4. Preheat the grill to high heat.
5. Grill the shrimp for 4 to 6 minutes, flipping the shrimp halfway through, or until the shrimp are pink on the outside and opaque in the center.
6. Serve hot.

Tip: You can try adding 1 tsp.—paprika to the marinade for added color and flavor. To save time, you can marinate the shrimp ahead of time.

Nutrition:

Calories: 401
Fat: 17.8g
Protein: 56.9g
Carbs: 3.9g

CHAPTER 6:

Poultry

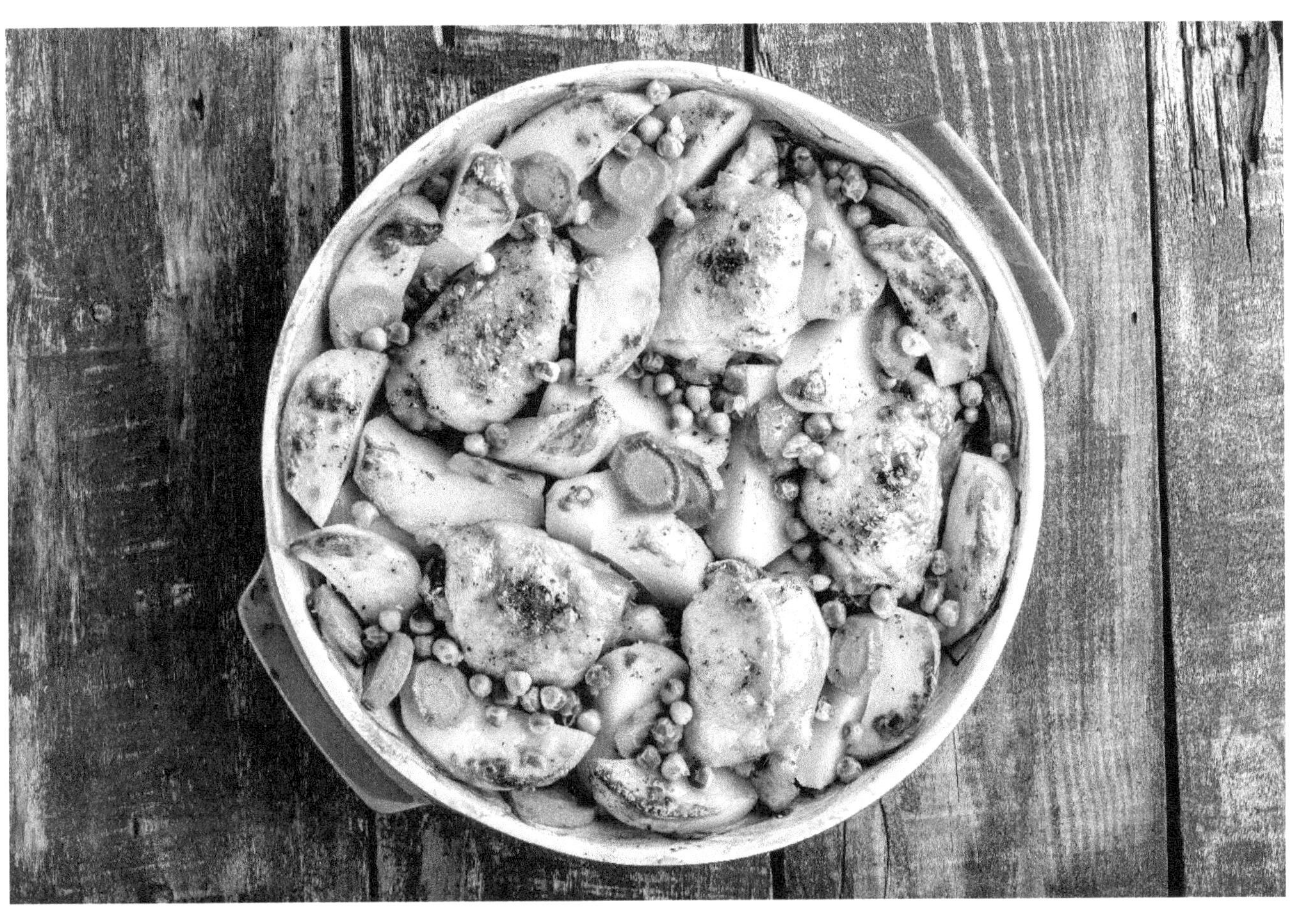

1. Turkey and Salsa Verde

Preparation Time: 5 minutes
Cooking Time: 50 minutes
Servings: 4

Ingredients:

- One big turkey breast, skinless, boneless, and cubed
- One and ½ cups Salsa Verde
- Salt and black pepper to the taste
- 1 tbsp. olive oil
- One and ½ cups feta cheese, crumbled
- ¼ cup cilantro, chopped

Directions:

1. In a roasting pan greased with the oil, combine the turkey with the salsa, salt, and pepper and bake 400 degrees F for 50 minutes.
2. Add the cheese and the cilantro, toss gently, divide everything between plates and serve.

Nutrition:
Calories 332
Fat 15.4 g
Fiber 10
Carbs 22.1
Protein 34.5

2. Chicken with Peas

Preparation Time: 5 minutes
Cooking Time: 30 minutes
Servings: 4

Ingredients:

- Four chicken fillets
- 1 tsp. cayenne pepper
- 1 tsp. salt
- 1 tbsp. mayonnaise
- 1 cup green peas
- ¼ cup of water
- One carrot, peeled, chopped

Directions:

1. Sprinkle the chicken fillet with cayenne pepper and salt.
2. Line the baking tray using foil and place chicken fillets in it.
3. Then brush the chicken with mayonnaise.
4. Add carrot and green peas.
5. Then add water and cover the ingredients with foil.
6. Bake the chicken for 30 minutes at 355F.

Nutrition:
Calories 329
Fat 12.3
Fiber 2.3
Carbs 7.9
Protein 44.4

3. Chicken Wrap

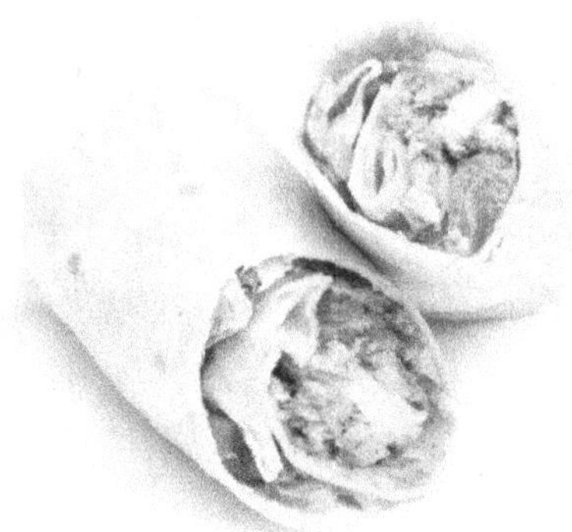

Preparation Time: 10 minutes
Cooking Time: 0 minutes
Servings: 2

Ingredients:

- Two whole wheat tortilla flatbreads
- Six chicken breast slices, skinless, boneless, cooked, and shredded
- A handful of baby spinach
- Two provolone cheese slices
- Four tomato slices
- Ten kalamata olives, pitted and sliced
- One red onion, sliced
- 2 tbsp. roasted peppers, chopped

Directions:

1. Arrange the tortillas on a working surface, and divide the chicken and the other ingredients on each.
2. Roll the tortillas and serve them right away.

Nutrition:
Calories 190
Fat 6.8 g Fiber 3.5 g

Carbs 15.1 g Protein 6.6 g

4. Almond Chicken Bites

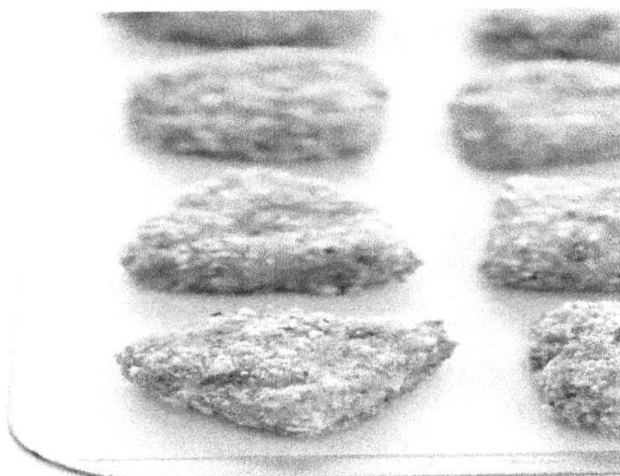

Preparation Time: 5 minutes
Cooking Time: 5 minutes
Servings: 8

Ingredients:

- 1-pound chicken fillet
- 1 tbsp. potato starch
- ½ tsp. salt
- 1 tsp. paprika
- 2 tbsp. wheat flour, whole grain
- One egg, beaten
- 1 tbsp. almond butter

Directions:

1. Chop the chicken fillet on the small pieces and place it in the bowl.
2. Add egg, salt, and potato starch. Mix up the chicken. Then mix up wheat flour and paprika. Then coat every chicken piece in wheat flour mixture.
3. Place almond butter in the skillet and heat it. Add chicken popcorn and roast it for 5 minutes over medium heat.
4. Dry the chicken popcorn with the help of a paper towel.

Nutrition:
Calories 141 Fat 5.9 g
Fiber 0.4 g Carbs 3.3 g Protein 17.8 g

5. Turkey, Artichokes and Asparagus

Preparation Time: 5 minutes
Cooking Time: 30 minutes
Serving: 4

Ingredients:

- Two turkey breasts, boneless, skinless, and halved
- 3 tbsp. olive oil
- One and ½ pounds asparagus, trimmed and halved
- 1 cup chicken stock
- A pinch of salt and black pepper
- 1 cup canned artichoke hearts, drained
- ¼ cup kalamata olives, pitted and sliced
- One shallot, chopped
- Three garlic cloves, minced
- 3 tbsp. dill, chopped

Directions:

1. Heat a pan with the oil over medium-high heat, add the turkey and the garlic, and brown for 4 minutes on each side.
2. Add the asparagus, the stock, and the rest of the ingredients except the dill, bring to a simmer and cook over medium heat for 20 minutes.
3. Add the dill, divide the mix between plates and serve.

Nutrition:
Calories 291
Fat 16 g
Fiber 10.3 g
Carbs 22.8 g
Protein 34.5 g

6. Garlic Chicken and Endives

Preparation Time: 5 minutes
Cooking Time: 15 minutes
Serving: 4

Ingredients:

- 1-pound chicken breasts, skinless, boneless, and cubed
- Two endives, sliced
- 2 tbsp. olive oil
- Four garlic cloves, minced
- ½ cup chicken stock
- 2 tbsp. parmesan, grated
- 1 tbsp. parsley, chopped
- Salt and black pepper to the taste

Directions:

1. Heat a pan with the oil over medium-high heat, add the chicken and cook for 5 minutes.
2. Add the endives, garlic, the stock, salt, and pepper, stir, bring to a simmer and cook over medium-high heat for 10 minutes.
3. Add the parmesan and the parsley, toss gently, divide everything between plates and serve.

Nutrition:

Calories 280
Fat 9.2g
Fiber 10.8g
Carbs 21.6g
Protein 33.8g

7. Butter Chicken Thighs

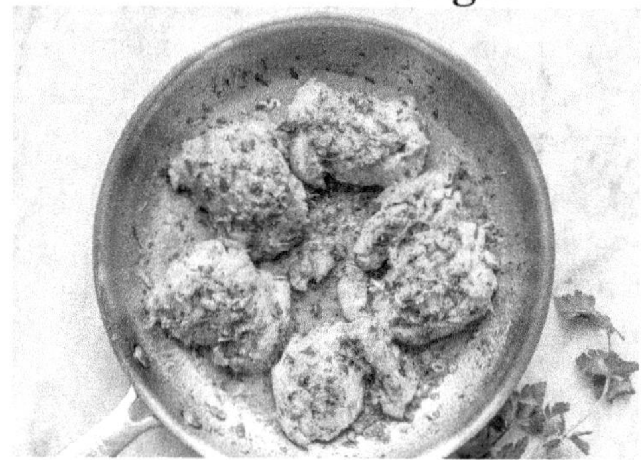

Preparation Time: 5 minutes
Cooking Time: 30 minutes
Serving: 4

Ingredients:

- 1 tsp. fennel seeds
- One garlic clove, peeled
- 1 tbsp. butter
- 1 tsp. coconut oil
- ¼ tsp. thyme
- ½ tsp. salt
- 1 oz. fennel bulb, chopped
- 1 oz. shallot, chopped
- Four chicken thighs, skinless, boneless
- 1 tsp. ground black pepper

Directions:

1. Rub the chicken thighs with ground black pepper.
2. In the skillet, mix up together butter and coconut oil.
3. Add fennel seeds, garlic clove, thyme, salt, and shallot.
4. Roast the mixture for 1 minute.
5. Then add fennel bulb and chicken thighs.
6. Roast the chicken thighs for 2 minutes from each side over high heat.
7. Then transfer the skillet with chicken in the oven and cook the meal for 20 minutes at 360F.

Nutrition:

Calories 324
Fat 14.9g
Fiber 0.6g
Carbs 2.6g
Protein 42.7g

8. Chicken and Olives Salsa

Preparation Time: 10 minutes
Cooking Time: 25 minutes
Serving: 4

Ingredients:

- 2 tbsp. avocado oil
- Four chicken breast halves, skinless and boneless
- Salt and black pepper to the taste
- 1 tbsp. sweet paprika
- One red onion, chopped
- 1 tbsp. balsamic vinegar
- 2 tbsp. parsley, chopped
- One avocado, peeled, pitted, and cubed
- 2 tbsp. black olives, pitted and chopped

Directions:

1. Heat and set your grill over medium-high heat, add the chicken brushed with half of the oil and seasoned with paprika, salt, and pepper, cook for 7 minutes on each side, and divide between plates.
2. Meanwhile, in a bowl, mix the onion with the rest of the ingredients and the remaining oil, toss, add on top of the chicken and serve.

Nutrition:

Calories 289
Fat 12.4g

Fiber 9.1g
Carbs 23.8g
Protein 14.3g

Fat 8
Fiber 2
Carbs 9
Protein 12

9. Chili Chicken Mix

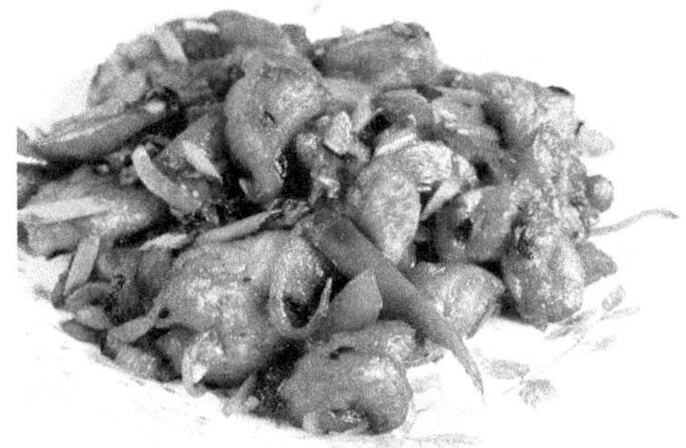

Preparation Time: 10 minutes
Cooking Time: 18 minutes
Serving: 4

Ingredients:

- 2 pounds chicken thighs, skinless and boneless
- 2 tbsp. olive oil
- 2 cups yellow onion, chopped
- 1 tsp. onion powder
- 1 tsp. smoked paprika
- 1 tsp. chili pepper
- ½ tsp. coriander seeds, ground
- 2 tsp. oregano, dried
- 2 tsp. parsley flakes
- 30 ounces canned tomatoes, chopped
- ½ cup black olives pitted and halved

Directions:

1. Set the instant pot on Sauté mode then add the oil, heat it, add the onion, onion powder, and the rest of the ingredients except the tomatoes, olives, and the chicken, stir, and sauté 10 minutes.
2. Add the chicken, tomatoes, and olives, put the lid on, and cook on High for 8 minutes.
3. Release the pressure naturally for 10 minutes, split the mix into bowls and serve.

Nutrition:

Calories 153

10. Duck and Orange Warm Salad

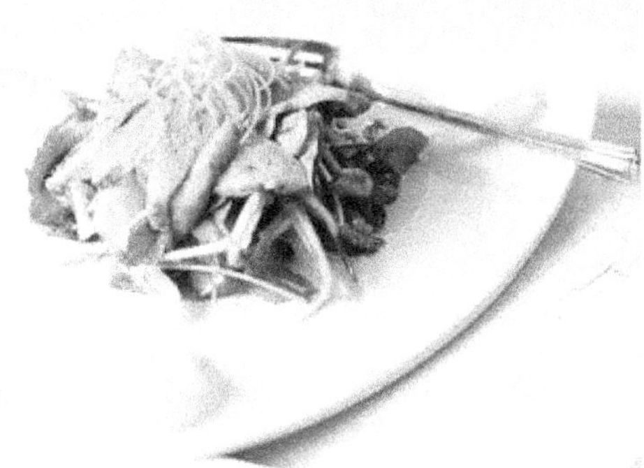

Preparation Time: 10 minutes
Cooking Time: 25 minutes
Serving: 4

Ingredients:

- 2 tbsp. balsamic vinegar
- Two oranges, peeled and cut into segments
- 1 tsp. orange zest, grated
- 1 tbsp. orange juice
- Three shallots, minced
- 2 tbsp. olive oil
- Salt and black pepper to the taste
- Two duck breasts, boneless and skin scored
- 2 cups baby arugula
- 2 tbsp. chives, chopped

Directions:

1. Heat a pan with the oil over medium-high heat, add the duck breasts skin side down, and brown for 5 minutes.
2. Flip the duck, add the shallot and the other ingredients except for the arugula, orange, and the chives, and cook for 15 minutes more.
3. Transfer the duck breasts to a cutting board, cool down, cut into strips, and put in a salad bowl.
4. Add the remaining ingredients, toss, and serve warm.

Nutrition:

Calories 304
Fat 15.4
Fiber 12.6
Carbs 25.1
Protein 36.4

11.   Turmeric Baked Chicken Breast

Preparation Time: 5 minutes
Cooking Time: 40 minutes
Serving: 2

Ingredients:

- 8 oz. chicken breast, skinless, boneless
- 2 tbsp. capers
- 1 tsp. olive oil
- ½ tsp. paprika
- ½ tsp. ground turmeric
- ½ tsp. salt
- ½ tsp. minced garlic

Directions:

1. Make the lengthwise cut in the chicken breast.
2. Rub the chicken with olive oil, paprika, capers, ground turmeric, salt, and minced garlic.
3. Then fill the chicken cut with capers and secure it with toothpicks.
4. Bake the chicken breast for 40 minutes at 350F.
5. Remove the toothpicks from the chicken breast and slice it.

Nutrition:
Calories 156
Fat 5.4 Fiber 0.6
Carbs 1.3
Protein 24.4

12.   Chicken Tacos

Preparation Time: 10 minutes
Cooking Time: 20 minutes
Servings: 4
Cooking Time: 20 Minutes

Ingredients:

- Two bread tortillas
- 1 tsp. butter
- 2 tsp. olive oil
- 1 tsp. Taco seasoning
- 6 oz. chicken breast, skinless, boneless, sliced
- 1/3 cup Cheddar cheese, shredded
- One bell pepper, cut on the wedges

Directions:

1. Pour 1 tsp. of olive oil in the skillet and add chicken.
2. Sprinkle the meat with Taco seasoning and mix up well.
3. Roast chicken for 10 minutes over medium heat. Stir it from time to time.
4. Then transfer the cooked chicken to the plate.
5. Add remaining olive oil to the skillet.
6. Then add bell pepper and roast it for 5 minutes. Stir it all the time.
7. Mix up together bell pepper with chicken.
8. Toss butter in the skillet and melt it.
9. Put one tortilla in the skillet.
10. Put Cheddar cheese on the tortilla and flatten it.
11. Then add a chicken-pepper mixture and cover it with the second tortilla.
12. Roast the quesadilla for 2 minutes from each side.
13. Cut the cooked meal on the halves and transfer it to the serving plates.

Nutrition:
Calories 194
Fat 8.3 g
Fiber 0.6 g
Carbs 16.4g
Protein 13.2 g

13.   Chicken and Butter Sauce

Preparation Time: 5 minutes
Cooking Time: 30 minutes
Serving: 5

Ingredients:

- 1-pound chicken fillet
- 1/3 cup butter, softened
- 1 tbsp. rosemary
- ½ tsp. thyme
- 1 tsp. salt

- ½ lemon

Directions:

1. Churn together thyme, salt, and rosemary.
2. Chop the chicken fillet roughly and mix it up with churned butter mixture.
3. Place the prepared chicken in the baking dish.
4. Squeeze the lemon over the chicken.
5. Chop the squeezed lemon and add it to the baking dish.
6. Cover the chicken with foil and bake it for 20 minutes at 365F.
7. Then discard the foil and bake the chicken for 10 minutes more.

Nutrition:
Calories 285
Fat 19.1
Fiber 0.5
Carbs 1
Protein 26.5

14.   Turkey and Cranberry Sauce

Preparation Time: 10 minutes
Cooking Time: 50 minutes
Serving: 4

Ingredients:

- 1 cup chicken stock
- 2 tbsp. avocado oil
- ½ cup cranberry sauce
- One big turkey breast, skinless, boneless, and sliced
- One yellow onion, roughly chopped
- Salt and black pepper to the taste

Directions:

1. Heat a pan with the avocado oil over medium-high heat, add the onion and sauté for 5 minutes.
2. Add the turkey and brown for 5 minutes more.
3. Add the rest of the ingredients, toss, introduce in the oven at 350 degrees F and cook for 40 minutes

Nutrition:
Calories 382
Fat 12.6

Fiber 9.6
Carbs 26.6
Protein 17.6

15.   Coriander and Coconut Chicken

Preparation Time: 10 minutes
Cooking Time: 30 minutes
Serving: 4

Ingredients:

- 2 pounds chicken thighs, skinless, boneless, and cubed
- 2 tbsp. olive oil
- Salt and black pepper to the taste
- 3 tbsp. coconut flesh, shredded
- One and ½ tsp. orange extract
- 1 tbsp. ginger, grated
- ¼ cup orange juice
- 2 tbsp. coriander, chopped
- 1 cup chicken stock
- ¼ tsp. red pepper flakes

Directions:

1. Heat a pan with the oil over medium-high heat, add the chicken, and brown for 4 minutes on each side.
2. Add salt, pepper, and the rest of the ingredients, bring to a simmer and cook over medium heat for 20 minutes.
3. Divide the mix between plates and serve hot.

Nutrition:
Calories 297,
Fat 14.4g
Fiber 9.6g
Carbs 22g
Protein 25g

16.   Chicken Pilaf

Preparation Time: 10 minutes
Cooking Time: 30 minutes
Serving: 4

Ingredients:

- 4 tbsp. avocado oil

- 2 pounds chicken breasts, skinless, boneless, and cubed
- ½ cup yellow onion, chopped
- Four garlic cloves, minced
- 8 ounces brown rice
- 4 cups chicken stock
- ½ cup kalamata olives pitted
- ½ cup tomatoes, cubed
- 6 ounces baby spinach
- ½ cup feta cheese, crumbled
- A pinch of salt and black pepper
- 1 tbsp. marjoram, chopped
- 1 tbsp. basil, chopped
- Juice of ½ lemon
- ¼ cup pine nuts, toasted

Directions:

1. Heat a pot with 1 tbsp. avocado oil set over medium-high heat, add the chicken, salt, and pepper, brown for 5 minutes on each side, and transfer to a bowl.
2. Heat the pot again with the rest of the avocado oil over medium heat, add the onion and garlic and sauté for 3 minutes.
3. Add the rice, the rest of the ingredients except the pine nuts, return the chicken, toss, bring it to a simmer and cook over medium heat for 20 minutes.
4. Divide the mix between plates, top each serving with some pine nuts and serve.

Nutrition:
Calories 283
Fat 12.5g
Fiber 8.2g
Carbs 21.5 g
Protein 13.4 g

17.   Chicken and Black Beans

Preparation Time: 10 minutes
Cooking Time: 20 minutes
Serving: 4
Cooking Time: 20 Minutes

Ingredients:

- 12 oz. chicken breast, skinless, boneless, chopped
- 1 tbsp. taco seasoning
- 1 tbsp. nut oil
- ½ tsp. cayenne pepper
- ½ tsp. salt
- ½ tsp. garlic, chopped
- ½ red onion, sliced
- 1/3 cup black beans, canned, rinsed
- ½ cup Mozzarella, shredded

Directions:

1. Rub the chopped chicken breast with taco seasoning, salt, and cayenne pepper.
2. Place the chicken in the skillet, add nut oil and roast it for 10 minutes over medium heat. Mix up the chicken pieces from time to time to avoid burning.
3. After this, transfer the chicken to the plate.
4. Add sliced onion and then garlic to the skillet. Roast the vegetables for 5 minutes. Stir them constantly. Then add black beans and stir well—Cook the ingredients for 2 minutes more.
5. Add the chopped chicken and mix up well. Top the meal with Mozzarella cheese.
6. Close the lid and cook the meal for 3 minutes.

Nutrition:
Calories 209
Fat 6.4
Fiber 2.8
Carbs 13.7, 22.7

18.   Coconut Chicken

Preparation Time: 10 minutes
Cooking Time: 5 minutes
Serving: 4

Ingredients:

- 6 oz. chicken fillet
- ¼ cup of sparkling water
- One egg
- 3 tbsp. coconut flakes
- 1 tbsp. coconut oil
- 1 tsp. Greek Seasoning

Directions:

1. Cut the chicken fillet into small pieces (nuggets).
2. Then crack the egg in the bowl and whisk it.
3. Mix up together egg and sparkling water.
4. Add Greek seasoning and stir gently.
5. Dip the chicken nuggets in the egg mixture and then coat in the coconut flakes.
6. Melt the coconut oil in the skillet and heat it until it is shimmering.
7. Then add prepared chicken nuggets.
8. Roast them for 1 minute from each or until they are light brown.
9. Dry the cooked chicken nuggets with the paper towels help and transfer them to the serving plates.

Nutrition:
Calories 141 Fat 8.9
Fiber 0.3 Carbs 1 Protein 13.9

19. Ginger Chicken Drumsticks

Preparation Time: 10 minutes
Cooking Time: 30 minutes
Serving: 4

Ingredients:

- Four chicken drumsticks
- One apple, grated
- 1 tbsp. curry paste
- 4 tbsp. milk
- 1 tsp. coconut oil
- 1 tsp. chili flakes
- ½ tsp. minced ginger

Directions:

1. Mix up together grated apple, curry paste, milk, chili flakes, and minced garlic.
2. Put coconut oil in the skillet and melt it.
3. Add apple mixture and stir well.
4. Then add chicken drumsticks and mix up well.
5. Roast the chicken for 2 minutes from each side.
6. Then preheat the oven to 360F.

7. Place the skillet with chicken drumsticks in the oven and bake for 25 minutes.

Nutrition:
Calories 150
Fat 6.4g
Fiber 1.4g
Carbs 9.7g
Protein 13.5 g

20. Parmesan Chicken

Preparation Time: 10 minutes
Cooking Time: 30 minutes
Serving: 3

Ingredients:

- 1-pound chicken breast, skinless, boneless
- 2 oz. Parmesan, grated
- 1 tsp. dried oregano
- ½ tsp. dried cilantro
- 1 tbsp. Panko bread crumbs
- One egg, beaten
- 1 tsp. turmeric

Directions:

1. Cut the chicken breast into three servings.
2. Then combine Parmesan, oregano, cilantro, bread crumbs, and turmeric.
3. Dip the chicken servings in the beaten egg carefully.
4. Then coat every chicken piece in the cheese-bread crumbs mixture.
5. Line the baking tray using the baking paper.
6. Arrange the chicken pieces in the tray.
7. Bake the chicken for 30 minutes at 365F.

Nutrition:
Calories 267 Fat 9.5
Fiber 0.5 Carbs 3.2 Protein 40.4

21. Chicken with Caper Sauce

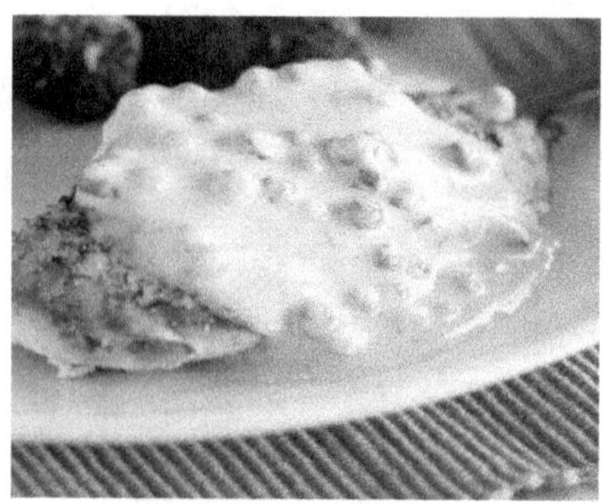

Preparation Time: 10 minutes
Cooking Time: 18 minutes
Serving: 5

Ingredients:

For Chicken:

- Two eggs
- Salt and ground black pepper, as required
- 1 cup dry breadcrumbs
- 2 tbsp. olive oil
- 1½ pounds skinless, boneless chicken breast halves, pounded into ¾inch thickness and cut into pieces

For Capers Sauce:

- 3 tbsp. capers
- ½ cup dry white wine
- 3 tbsp. fresh lemon juice
- Salt and ground black pepper, as required
- 2 tbsp. fresh parsley, chopped

Directions:

1. For the chicken: in a shallow dish, add the eggs, salt, and black pepper and beat until well combined.
2. In another shallow dish, place breadcrumbs. Soak the chicken pieces in an egg mixture, then coat with the breadcrumbs evenly.
3. Shake off the excess breadcrumbs.
4. Cook the oil over medium heat and cook the chicken pieces for about 5-7 minutes per side or desired doneness.
5. With a slotted spoon, situate the chicken pieces onto a paper towel-lined plate. With a portion of the foil, cover the chicken pieces to keep them warm.
6. In the same skillet, incorporate all the sauce ingredients except parsley and cook for about 2-3 minutes, stirring

continuously. Mix in the parsley and remove from heat. Serve the chicken pieces with the topping of capers sauce.

Nutrition:

Calories 352

Fat 13.5g

Carbs 2g

Protein 1.2g

22. Turkey Burgers with Mango Salsa

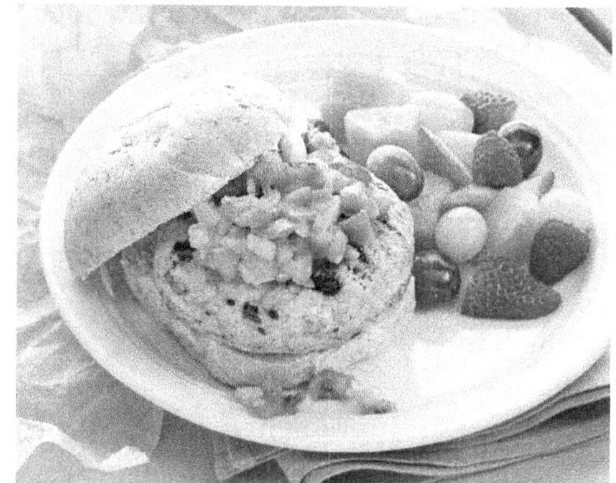

Preparation Time: 15 minutes
Cooking Time: 10 minutes
Serving: 6

Ingredients:

- 1½ pounds ground turkey breast
- 1 tsp. sea salt, divided
- ¼ tsp. freshly ground black pepper
- 2 tbsp. extra-virgin olive oil
- Two mangos, peeled, pitted, and cubed
- ½ red onion, finely chopped
- Juice of 1 lime
- One garlic clove, minced
- ½ jalapeño pepper, seeded and finely minced
- 2 tbsp. chopped fresh cilantro leaves

Directions:

1. Form the turkey breast into four patties

and season with ½ tsp. of sea salt and the pepper.

2. Cook the olive oil in a nonstick skillet until it shimmers. Add the turkey patties and cook for about 5 minutes per side until browned.

3. While the patties cook, mix the mango, red onion, lime juice, garlic, jalapeño, cilantro, and remaining ½ tsp. of sea salt in a small bowl. Spoon the salsa over the turkey patties and serve.

Nutrition

Calories 384 Fat 3g

Carbs 27g Protein 34g

23. Chicken Sausage and Peppers

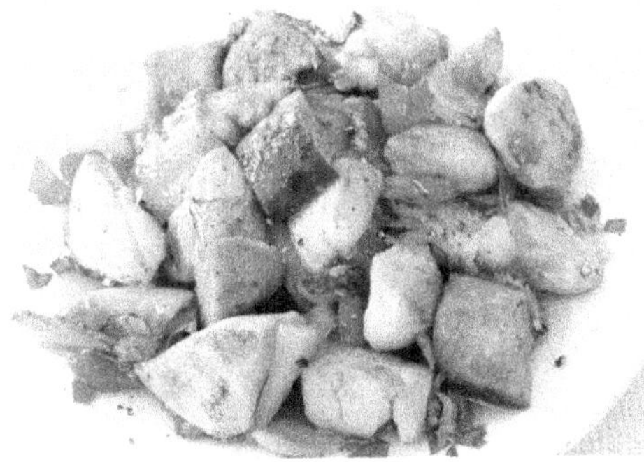

Preparation Time: 10 minutes

Cooking Time: 20 minutes

Serving: 6

Ingredients:

- 2 tbsp. extra-virgin olive oil
- 6 Italian chicken sausage links
- One onion
- One red bell pepper
- One green bell pepper
- Three garlic cloves, minced
- ½ cup dry white wine
- ½ tsp. sea salt
- ¼ tsp. freshly ground black pepper
- Pinch red pepper flakes

Directions:

1. Cook the olive oil on a large skillet until it shimmers.

2. Add the sausages and cook for 5 to 7 minutes, occasionally turning, until browned and they reach an internal temperature of 165°F.

3. With tongs, remove the sausage from the pan and set it aside on a platter, tented with aluminum foil to keep warm.

4. Return the skillet to heat and mix in the onion, red bell pepper, and green bell pepper. Cook and occasionally stir until the vegetables begin to brown. Put in the garlic and cook for 30 seconds, stirring constantly.

5. Stir in the wine, sea salt, pepper, and red pepper flakes.

6. Pull out and fold in any browned bits from the bottom of the pan. Simmer for about 4 minutes more, stirring, until the liquid reduces by half. Spoon the peppers over the sausages and serve.

Nutrition:

Calories 173 Fat 1g

Carbs 6g Protein 22g

24. Chicken Piccata

Preparation Time: 10 minutes

Cooking Time: 15 minutes

Serving: 6

Ingredients:

- ½ cup whole-wheat flour
- ½ tsp. sea salt
- 1/8 tsp. freshly ground black pepper
- 1½ pounds chicken breasts, cut into six pieces
- 3 tbsp. extra-virgin olive oil
- 1 cup unsalted chicken broth
- ½ cup dry white wine
- Juice of 1 lemon
- Zest of 1 lemon
- ¼ cup capers drained and rinsed
- ¼ cup chopped fresh parsley leaves

Directions:

1. In a shallow dish, whisk the flour, sea salt, and pepper. Scour the chicken in the flour and tap off any excess. Cook the olive oil until it shimmers.

2. Put the chicken and cook for about 4 minutes per side until browned. Pull out the chicken from the pan and set it aside, tented with aluminum foil to keep warm.

3. Situate the skillet back to the heat and stir in the broth, wine, lemon juice, lemon zest, and capers. Use the side of a spoon scoop and fold in any browned bits from the pan's bottom.

4. Simmer until the liquid thickens. Take out the skillet from the heat and take the chicken back to the pan. Turn to coat. Stir in the parsley and serve.

Nutrition:
Calories 153 Fat 2g
Carbs 9g Protein 8g

25. One-Pan Tuscan Chicken

Preparation Time: 10 minutes
Cooking Time: 25 minutes
Serving: 6

Ingredients:

- ¼ cup extra-virgin olive oil, divided
- 1-pound boneless, skinless chicken breasts, cut into ¾-inch pieces
- One onion, chopped
- One red bell pepper, chopped
- Three garlic cloves, minced
- ½ cup dry white wine
- 1 (14-ounce) can crushed tomatoes, undrained
- 1 (14-ounce) can chopped tomatoes, drained
- 1 (14-ounce) can white beans, drained
- 1 tbsp. dried Italian seasoning
- ½ tsp. sea salt
- 1/8 tsp. freshly ground black pepper
- 1/8 tsp. red pepper flakes
- ¼ cup chopped fresh basil leaves

Directions:

1. Cook 2 tbsp. of olive oil until it shimmers. Mix in the chicken and cook until browned.

2. Remove the chicken from the skillet and set it aside on a platter, tented with aluminum foil to keep warm.

3. Situate the skillet back to heat and heat the remaining olive oil.

4. Add the onion and red bell pepper. Cook and rarely stir until the vegetables are soft.

5. Put the garlic and cook for 30 seconds, stirring constantly.

6. Stir in the wine, and use the spoon's side to scoop out any browned bits from the bottom of the pan. Cook for 1 minute, stirring.

7. Mix in the crushed and chopped tomatoes, white beans, Italian seasoning, sea salt, pepper, and red pepper flakes.

8. Allow simmering. Cook for 5 minutes, stirring occasionally.

9. Put the chicken back and any juices that have collected into the skillet. Cook until the chicken is cook through.

10. Take out from the heat and stir in the basil before serving.

Nutrition:
Calories 271
Fat 8g
Carbs 29g
Protein 14g

26. Spinach and Feta–Stuffed Chicken Breasts

Preparation Time: 10 minutes
Cooking Time: 45 minutes
Serving: 4

Ingredients:

- 2 tbsp. extra-virgin olive oil
- 1-pound fresh baby spinach
- Three garlic cloves, minced
- Zest of 1 lemon
- ½ tsp. sea salt
- 1/8 tsp. freshly ground black pepper
- ½ cup crumbled feta cheese
- Four boneless, skinless chicken breasts

Directions:

1. Preheat the oven to 350°F. Cook the olive oil over medium heat until it shimmers. Add the spinach. Continue cooking and stirring until wilted.
2. Stir in the garlic, lemon zest, sea salt, and pepper. Cook for 30 seconds, stirring constantly. Cool slightly and mix in the cheese.
3. Spread the spinach and cheese mixture in an even layer over the chicken pieces and roll the breast around the filling.
4. Hold closed with toothpicks or butcher's twine.
5. Place the breasts in a 9-by-13-inch baking dish and bake for 30 to 40 minutes, or until the chicken have an internal temperature of 165°F.
6. Take out from the oven and set aside for 5 minutes before slicing and serving.

Nutrition

Calories 263

Fat 3g

Carbs 7g

Protein 17g

27.　Rosemary　Baked　Chicken Drumsticks

Preparation Time: 5 minutes

Cooking Time: 60 minutes

Serving: 4

Ingredients:

- 2 tbsp. chopped fresh rosemary leaves
- 1 tsp. garlic powder
- ½ tsp. sea salt
- 1/8 tsp. freshly ground black pepper
- Zest of 1 lemon
- 12 chicken drumsticks

Directions:

1. Preheat the oven to 350°F. Mix the rosemary, garlic powder, sea salt, pepper, and lemon zest.
2. Situate the drumsticks in a 9-by-13-inch baking dish and sprinkle with the rosemary mixture.
3. Bake until the chicken reaches an internal temperature of 165°F.

Nutrition:

Calories 163

Fat 1g

Carbs 2g

Protein 26g

28.　Chicken with Onions, Potatoes, Figs, and Carrots

Preparation Time: 45 minutes

Cooking Time: 5 minutes

Serving: 4

Ingredients:

- 2 cups fingerling potatoes, halved
- Four fresh figs, quartered
- Two carrots, julienned
- 2 tbsp. extra-virgin olive oil
- 1 tsp. sea salt, divided
- ¼ tsp. freshly ground black pepper
- Four chicken leg-thigh quarters
- 2 tbsp. chopped fresh parsley leaves

Directions:

1. Preheat the oven to 425°F.
2. In a small bowl, toss the potatoes, figs, and carrots with the olive oil, ½ tsp., sea salt, and pepper. Spread in a 9-by-13-inch baking dish.
3. Season, the chicken with the rest of t sea salt. Place it on top of the vegetables.
4. Bake until the vegetables are soft and the chicken reaches an internal temperature of 165°F. Sprinkle with the parsley and serve.

Nutrition:

Calories 429

Fat 4g

Carbs 27g

Protein 52g

29.　Moussaka

Preparation Time: 10 minutes

Cooking Time: 45 minutes

Serving: 8

Ingredients:

- 5 tbsp. extra-virgin olive oil, divided
- One eggplant, sliced (unpeeled)

- One onion, chopped
- One green bell pepper, seeded and chopped
- 1-pound ground turkey
- Three garlic cloves, minced
- 2 tbsp. tomato paste
- 1 (14-ounce) can chopped tomatoes, drained
- 1 tbsp. Italian seasoning
- 2 tsp. Worcestershire sauce
- 1 tsp. dried oregano
- ½ tsp. ground cinnamon
- 1 cup unsweetened nonfat plain Greek yogurt
- One egg, beaten
- ¼ tsp. freshly ground black pepper
- ¼ tsp. ground nutmeg
- ¼ cup grated Parmesan cheese
- 2 tbsp. chopped fresh parsley leaves

Directions:

1. Preheat the oven to 400°F. Cook 3 tbsp. of olive oil until it shimmers.
2. Add the eggplant slices and brown for 3 to 4 minutes per side.
3. Transfer to paper towels to drain.
4. Return the skillet to heat and pour the remaining 2 tbsp. of olive oil. Add the onion and green bell pepper.
5. Continue cooking until the vegetables are soft. Remove from the pan and set aside.
6. Pull out the skillet to the heat and stir in the turkey.
7. Cook for about 5 minutes, crumbling with a spoon until browned.
8. Stir in the garlic and cook for 30 seconds, stirring constantly.
9. Stir in the tomato paste, tomatoes, Italian seasoning, Worcestershire sauce, oregano, and cinnamon.
10. Place the onion and bell pepper back to the pan. Cook for 5 minutes, stirring. Combine the yogurt, egg, pepper, nutmeg, and cheese.
11. Arrange half of the meat mixture in a 9-by-13-inch baking dish.
12. Layer with half the eggplant. Add the remaining meat mixture and the remaining eggplant.
13. Spread with the yogurt mixture.
14. Bake until golden brown. Garnish with the parsley and serve.

Nutrition:

Calories 338

Fat 5g

Carbs 14g

Protein 28g

30.   Seasoned Buttered Chicken

Preparation Time: 10 minutes

Cooking Time: 25 minutes

Serving: 4

Ingredients:

- ½ c. Heavy Whipping Cream
- 1 tbsp. Salt
- ½ c. Bone Broth
- 1 tbsp. Pepper
- 4 tbsps. Butter
- 4 Chicken Breast Halves

Directions:

1. Place cooking pan on your oven over medium heat and add in one tbsp. of butter.
2. Once the butter is warm and melted, place the chicken in and cook for five minutes on either side.
3. At the end of this time, the chicken should be cooked through and golden; if it is, go ahead and place it on a plate.
4. Next, you are going to add the bone broth into the warm pan. Add heavy whipping cream, salt, and pepper.
5. Then, leave the pan alone until your sauce begins to simmer. Allow this process to happen for five minutes to let the sauce thicken up.
6. Finally, you will add the rest of your butter and the chicken back into the pan.
7. Be sure to use a spoon to place the sauce over your chicken and smother it completely. Serve

Nutrition:

Calories 350
Fat 25g
Carbs 10g
Protein 25g

31.　Double Cheesy Bacon Chicken

Preparation Time: 10 minutes
Cooking Time: 30 minutes
Serving: 4

Ingredients:

- 4 oz. or 113 g. Cream Cheese
- 1 c. Cheddar Cheese
- 8 strips Bacon
- Sea salt
- Pepper
- 2 Garlic cloves, finely chopped
- Chicken Breast
- 1 tbsp. Bacon Grease or Butter

Directions:

1. Ready the oven to 400°F. Slice the chicken breasts in half to make them thin
2. Season with salt, pepper, and garlic. Grease a baking pan with butter and place chicken breasts into it.
3. Add the cream cheese and cheddar cheese on top of the breasts
4. Add bacon slices as well. Place the pan in the oven for 30 minutes and serve hot

Nutrition:
Calories 610
Fat 32g

Carbs 3g
Protein 37g

32.　Crispy Italian Chicken

Preparation Time: 10 minutes
Cooking Time: 30 minutes
Serving: 4

Ingredients:

- Four chicken legs
- 1 tsp. dried basil
- 1 tsp. dried oregano
- Salt and pepper
- 3 tbsps. olive oil
- 1 tbsp. balsamic vinegar

Directions:

1. Season the chicken well with basil and oregano. Using a skillet, add oil and heat. Add the chicken to the hot oil.
2. Let each side cook for 5 minutes until golden, then cover the skillet with a lid.
3. Adjust your heat to medium and cook for 10 minutes on one side, then flip the chicken repeatedly, cooking for another 10 minutes until crispy.
4. Serve the chicken and enjoy.

Nutrition:
Calories 262
Fat 14g
Carbs 11g
Protein 32.6g

CHAPTER 7:

Snack and Appetizer

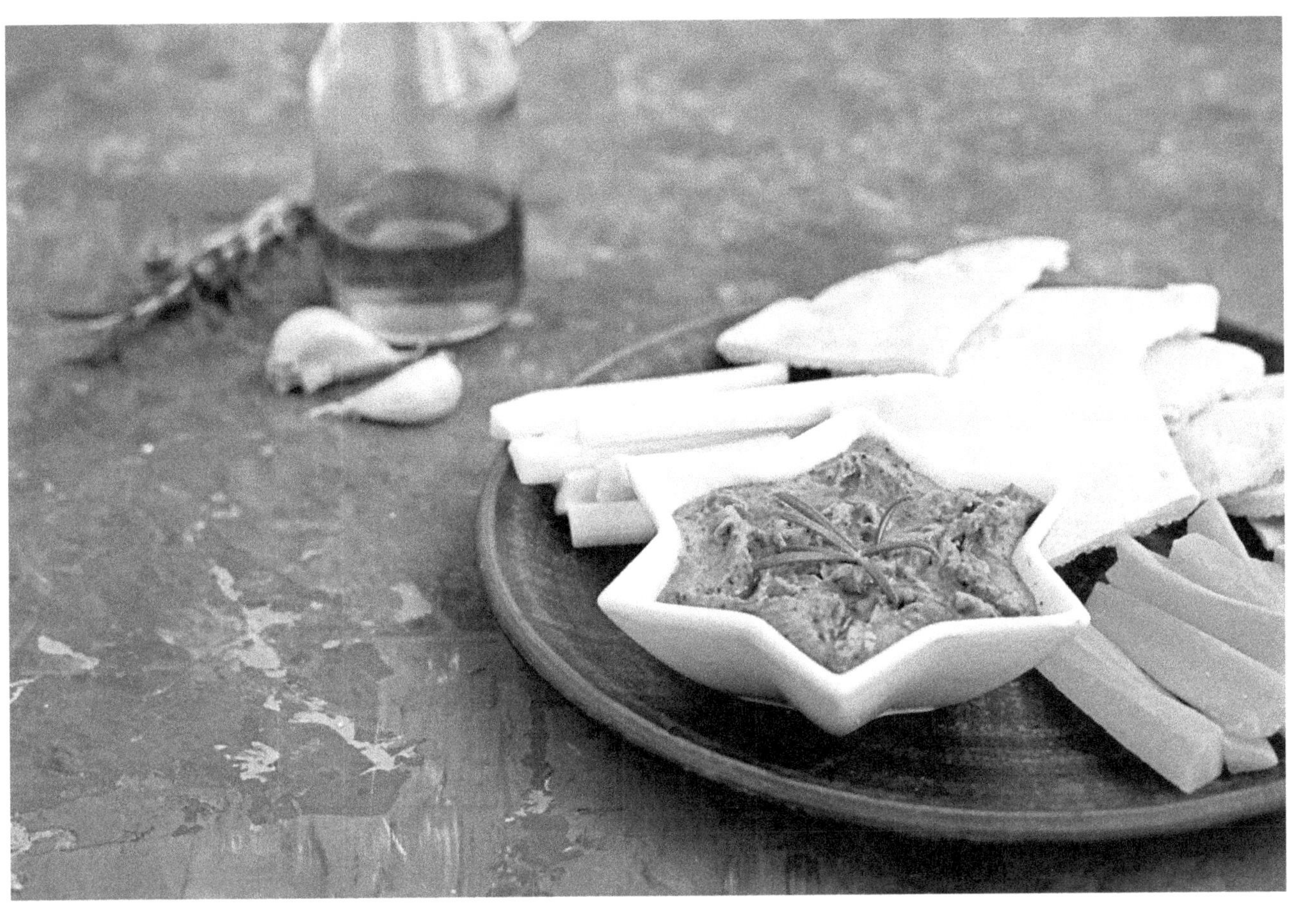

1. Flavorful Italian Peppers

Preparation Time: 10 minutes
Cooking Time: 3 minutes
Serving: 4

Ingredients:

- Four red bell peppers, cut into strips and remove seeds
- 1/2 tsp. Italian seasoning
- 1/2 tsp. garlic powder
- 1 tbsp. vinegar
- 3 tbsp. olive oil
- 1 cup of water Pepper
- Salt

Directions:

1. Add bell peppers and water into the instant pot.
2. Seal pot with lid and cook on high for 3 minutes.
3. Once done, release pressure using quick release. Remove lid.
4. In a prepared small bowl, mix oil, vinegar, garlic powder, Italian seasoning, pepper, and salt.
5. Once bell peppers are cooked, then pour oil mixture over bell peppers and mix well.
6. Serve warm and enjoy.

Nutrition:
Calories 132
Fat 11 g
Carbohydrates 9.4 g
Sugar 6.2 g
Protein 1.3 g
Cholesterol 0 mg

2. Spicy Jalapeno Spinach Artichoke Dip

Preparation Time: 10 minutes
Cooking Time: 3 minutes
Serving: 15

Ingredients:

- 10 oz. spinach, chopped
- 1/2 cup parmesan cheese, grated
- 8 oz. Italian cheese, shredded
- 1/4 cup fresh parsley, chopped
- 2 tbsp. jalapeno, diced
- 1/2 tbsp. garlic, minced
- tbsp. green onion, chopped
- 14 oz. cream cheese, cubed
- 18 oz. jar marinated artichoke hearts, chopped
- 1 1/2 tbsp. fresh lemon juice
- 1/2 cup vegetable stock

Directions:

1. Add all ingredients except parmesan cheese and Italian cheese into the instant pot and stir well.
2. Seal pot with lid and cook on high for 3 minutes.
3. If it is done, release pressure naturally for 5 minutes, and then release remaining using quick release. Remove lid.
4. Set pot on sauté mode. Add parmesan cheese and Italian cheese and stir well and cook until cheese is melted.
5. Serve and enjoy.

Nutrition:
Calories 195 Fat 16.3 g
Carbohydrates 3.7 g
Sugar 0.6 g
Protein 6.7 g
Cholesterol 42 mg

3. Pinto Bean Dip

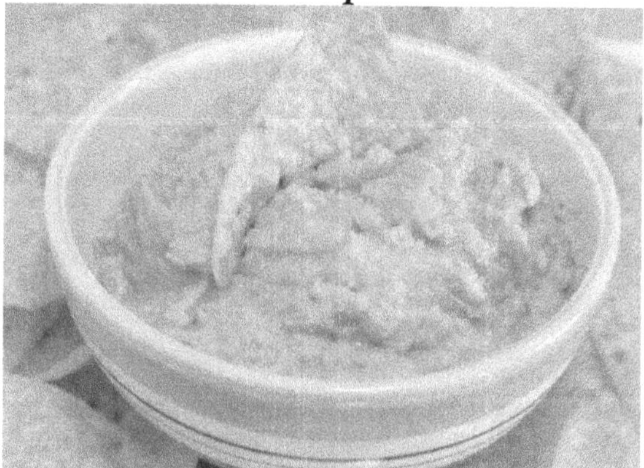

Preparation Time: 10 minutes
Cooking Time: 45 minutes
Serving: 6

Ingredients:

- 1 cup dry pinto beans
- 2 tsp. chili powder

- Three chilies de Arbol, remove the stem
- 4 cups of water
- 1 tsp. salt

Directions:
1. Add beans, chilies, and water into the instant pot and stir well.
2. Seal pot with lid and cook on high for 45 minutes.
3. If it is done, release pressure naturally for 10 minutes, and then release remaining using quick release. Remove lid.
4. Transfer instant pot bean mixture into the blender along with chili powder and salt and blend until smooth.
5. Serve and enjoy.

Nutrition:
Calories 139
Fat 0.6 g
Carbohydrates 24.6 g
Protein 8 g

4. Light & Creamy Garlic Hummus

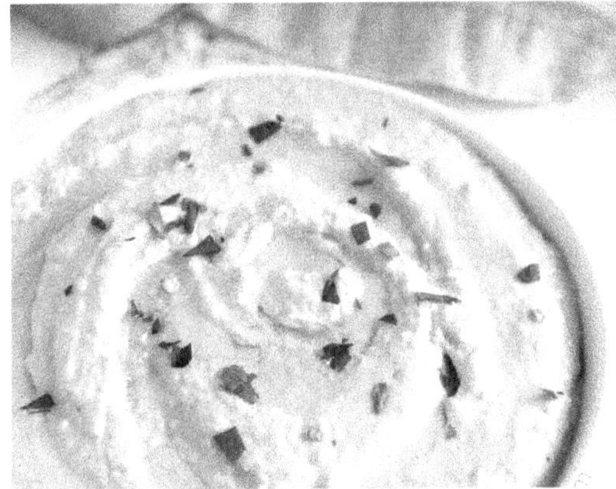

Preparation Time: 10 minutes
Cooking Time: 40 minutes
Serving: 12

Ingredients:
- 1 1/2 cups dry chickpeas, rinsed
- 2 1/2 tbsp. fresh lemon juice
- 1 tbsp. garlic, minced 1/2 cup tahini
- 6 cups of water Pepper
- Salt

Directions:
1. Add water and chickpeas into the instant pot.

2. Seal pot with a lid and select manual, and set timer for 40 minutes.
3. Once done, allow to release pressure naturally. Remove lid.
4. Drain chickpeas well and reserved 1/2 cup chickpeas liquid.
5. Transfer chickpeas, reserved liquid, lemon juice, garlic, tahini, pepper, and salt into the food processor and process until smooth.
6. Serve and enjoy.

Nutrition:
Calories 152
Fat 6.9 g
Carbohydrates 17.6 g
Sugar 2.8 g
Protein 6.6 g

5. Tasty Black Bean Dip

Preparation Time: 10 minutes
Cooking Time: 18 minutes
Servings: 6

Ingredients:
- 2 cups of dry black beans, soaked overnight, and drained
- 1 1/2 cups cheese, shredded
- 1 tsp. dried oregano
- 1/2 tsp. chili powder
- 2 cups tomatoes, chopped
- 2 tbsp. olive oil
- 1 1/2 tbsp. garlic, minced one medium onion, sliced
- 4 cups vegetable stock Pepper
- Salt

Directions:
1. Add all ingredients except cheese into the instant pot.
2. Seal pot with lid and cook on high for 18 minutes.
3. Once done, allow to release pressure naturally. Remove lid. Drain excess water.
4. Add cheese and stir until cheese is melted.
5. Blend bean mixture using an immersion blender until smooth.

6. Serve and enjoy.

Nutrition:
Calories 402
Fat 15.3 g
Carbohydrates 46.6 g
Sugar 4.4 g
Protein 22.2 g

6. Cucumber Tomato Okra Salsa

Preparation Time: 10 minutes
Cooking Time: 15 minutes
Servings: 4

Ingredients:

- 1 lb. tomatoes, chopped
- 1/4 tsp. red pepper flakes
- 1/4 cup fresh lemon juice
- One cucumber, chopped
- 1 tbsp. fresh oregano, chopped
- 1 tbsp. fresh basil, chopped
- 1 tbsp. olive oil
- One onion, chopped
- 1 tbsp. garlic, chopped
- 1/2 cups okra, chopped
- Pepper
- Salt

Directions:

1. Add oil into the inner pot of the instant pot and set the pot on sauté mode.
2. Add onion, garlic, pepper, and salt and sauté for 3 minutes.
3. Add remaining ingredients except for cucumber and stir well.
4. Seal pot with lid and cook on high for 12 minutes.
5. If it is done, release pressure naturally for 10 minutes, then release remaining using quick release. Remove lid.
6. Once the salsa mixture is cool, then add cucumber and mix well.
7. Serve and enjoy.

Nutrition:
Calories 99
Fat 4.2 g
Carbohydrates 14.3 g
Sugar 6.4 g
Protein 2.9 g

7. Cheesy Corn Dip

Preparation Time: 10 minutes
Cooking Time: 10 minutes
Servings: 6

Ingredients:

- Four ears corn
- 1/4 cup fresh basil, minced
- 1/4 cup fresh cilantro, minced
- 1 tbsp. fresh lime juice
- 1/4 tsp. cayenne
- 1/2 tsp. cumin
- 1/2 tsp. garlic powder
- 1 tsp. paprika
- 1 1/2 tsp. chili powder
- 1/4 cup mayonnaise
- 4 oz. cream cheese
- 1 cup of water
- Pepper
- Salt

Directions:

1. Pour water into the instant pot, then place the trivet in the pot.
2. Place corn on top of the trivet.
3. Seal pot with lid and cook on high for 5 minutes.
4. Once done, release pressure using quick release. Remove lid.
5. Remove corn and drain water from instant pot and clean the pot.
6. Cut corn from the cob. Add corn kernels, cayenne, cumin, garlic, paprika, chili powder, mayonnaise, cream cheese, pepper, and salt into the instant pot and stir well.
7. Seal pot with lid and cook on high for 5 minutes.
8. Once done, release pressure using quick release. Remove lid.
9. Add basil, cilantro, and lime juice and stir well.
10. Serve and enjoy.

Nutrition:
Calories 199
Fat 11.3 g

Carbohydrates 23.7 g

Sugar 4.3 g

Protein 5.1 g

8. Cheese Stuff Artichokes

Preparation Time: 10 minutes

Cooking Time: 20 minutes

Servings: 2

Ingredients:

- Two artichokes, trimmed and cut the 1/2-inch top
- 1/4 cup sour cream
- 1 tbsp. olive oil
- 1/4 cup fresh lemon juice
- 1 1/2 tsp. garlic, minced
- 1 tsp. Italian seasoning
- 1/2 cup parmesan cheese, grated
- 1 cup whole wheat breadcrumbs, homemade

Directions:

1. Spread artichoke leaves and clean the central core.
2. In a bowl, mix breadcrumbs, garlic, parmesan cheese, sour cream, oil, lemon juice, and Italian seasoning.
3. Stuff breadcrumbs mixture into the artichokes.
4. Pour 1 1/2 cup of water into the instant pot, then place the trivet in the pot.
5. Place artichokes on top of the trivet.
6. Seal pot with lid and cook on high for 20 minutes.
7. Once done, release pressure using quick release. Remove lid.
8. Serve and enjoy.

Nutrition:

Calories 428

Fat 20 g

Carbohydrates 48.7 g

Sugar 3.5 g

Protein 19.8 g

9. Flavorful Roasted Baby Potatoes

Preparation Time: 10 minutes

Cooking Time: 10 minutes

Servings: 4

Ingredients:

- 2 lbs. baby potatoes, clean and cut in half
- 1/2 cup vegetable stock
- 2 tsp. paprika
- 3/4 tsp. garlic powder
- 1 tsp. onion powder
- 1 tsp. Italian seasoning
- 1 tbsp. olive oil
- Pepper
- Salt

Directions:

1. Add oil into the inner pot of instant pot and set the pot on sauté mode.
2. Add potatoes and sauté for 5 minutes. Add remaining ingredients and stir well.
3. Seal pot with lid and cook on high for 5 minutes.
4. Once done, release pressure using quick release. Remove lid.
5. Stir well and serve.

Nutrition:

Calories 175 Fat 4.5 g

Carbohydrates 29.8 g Sugar 0.7 g

Protein 6.1 g

10. Rosemary Hummus

Preparation Time: 10 minutes

Cooking Time: 35 minutes

Servings: 10

Ingredients:

- 1 1/2 cups dry chickpeas
- 5 tbsp. rosemary garlic olive oil
- 1/2 tsp. smoked paprika
- 2 tbsp. fresh lemon juice
- 2 tbsp. tahini
- 6 cups of water
- 1 tsp. salt

Directions:

1. Add water and chickpeas into the instant pot.
2. Seal pot with lid and cook on high for 35 minutes.
3. If it is already done, release pressure naturally for 10 minutes, then release

remaining using quick release. Remove lid.

4. Drain chickpeas well and transfer into the food processor along with remaining ingredients and process until smooth.

5. Serve and enjoy.

Nutrition:
Calories 183
Fat 5 g
Carbohydrates 28 g
Sugar 3.5 g
Protein 7.3 g

11. Sausage Queso Dip

Preparation Time: 10 minutes
Cooking Time: 18 minutes
Servings: 8
Ingredients:

- 1 lb. Italian sausage, crumbled
- 4 cups Monterey jack cheese, shredded
- 12oz. milk
- 1/4 cup pickles peppers, diced
- 3.5oz. can olives, drained and sliced
- 14.5oz. can tomatoes, diced one small onion, chopped

Directions:

1. Set instant pot on sauté mode. Add sausage to the pot and cook for 3 minutes.
2. Add onion and sauté for 5 minutes.
3. Add remaining ingredients except for cheese and stir well and cook for 5 minutes.
4. Add shredded cheese and cook for 5 minutes or until cheese is melted.
5. Stir everything well and serve.

Nutrition:
Calories 458 Fat 35.8 g
Carbohydrates 6.8 g Sugar 4.4 g
Protein 27.1 g

12. Spicy Pepper Eggplant Spread

Preparation Time: 10 minutes
Cooking Time: 9 minutes
Servings: 4

Ingredients:

- 3 cups Italian eggplants, cut into 1/-inch chunks
- 1/2 cup tomatoes, diced
- 1 cup red pepper, diced
- 1/2 tsp. red pepper flakes
- 1 tbsp. vinegar
- 1 tbsp. garlic, minced
- 1/2 cup onion, diced
- 2 tbsp. olive oil
- 1/4 cup water
- 1 tsp. kosher salt

Directions:

1. Add oil into the inner pot of the instant pot and set the pot on sauté mode.
2. Add red pepper and eggplant and sauté for 5 minutes.
3. Add remaining ingredients and stir everything well.
4. Seal pot with lid and cook on high for 4 minutes.
5. Once done, release pressure using quick release. Remove lid.
6. Mash the spread mixture using the spatula and serve.

Nutrition:
Calories 237
Fat 19.2 g
Carbohydrates 18 g
Sugar 2.8 g
Protein 1 g

13. Garlic Pinto Bean Dip

Preparation Time: 10 minutes
Cooking Time: 43 minutes
Servings: 6

Ingredients:

- 1 cup dry pinto beans, rinsed
- 1/2 tsp. cumin
- 1/2 cup salsa two garlic cloves
- chipotle peppers in adobo sauce
- 5 cups vegetable stock
- Pepper Salt

Directions:

1. Add beans, stock, garlic, and chipotle peppers into the instant pot.
2. Seal pot with lid and cook on high for 43 minutes.
3. Once done, release pressure using quick release. Remove lid.
4. Drain beans well and reserve 1/2 cup of stock.
5. Transfer beans, reserve stock, and remaining ingredients into the food processor, and process until smooth.
6. Serve and enjoy.

Nutrition

Calories 129

Fat 0.9 g

Carbohydrates 23 g Sugar 1.9 g Protein 8 g

14. Creamy Potato Spread

Preparation Time: 10 minutes
Cooking Time: 15 minutes
Servings: 6

Ingredients:

- 1 lb. sweet potatoes, peeled and chopped
- 3/4 tbsp. fresh chives, chopped
- 1/2 tsp. paprika
- 1 tbsp. garlic, minced
- 1 cup tomatoes puree Pepper
- Salt

Directions:

1. Add all ingredients except chives into the inner pot of instant pot and stir well.
2. Seal pot with lid and cook on high for 15 minutes.
3. If it is already done, release pressure naturally for 10 minutes, then release remaining using quick release. Remove lid.
4. Transfer instant pot sweet potato mixture into the food processor and process until smooth.
5. Garnish with chives and serve.

Nutrition:

Calories 108 Fat 0.3 g

Carbohydrates 25.4 g Sugar 2.4 g

Protein 2 g

15. Slow-Cooked Cheesy Artichoke Dip

Preparation Time: 10 minutes
Cooking Time: 60 minutes
Servings: 6

Ingredients:

- 10 Oz can artichoke hearts, drained and chopped
- 4 cups spinach, chopped
- 8 oz. cream cheese
- 3 tbsp. sour cream 1/4 cup mayonnaise
- 3/4 cup mozzarella cheese, shredded
- 1/4 cup parmesan cheese, grated
- Three garlic cloves, minced
- 1/2 tsp. dried parsley Pepper
- Salt

Directions:

1. Put all ingredients inside the inner pot of the instant pot and then stir well.
2. Seal the pot with the lid, select slow cook mode, and set the timer for 60 minutes. Stir once while cooking.
3. Serve and enjoy.

Nutrition:

Calories 226

Fat 19.3 g

Carbohydrates 7.5 g

Sugar 1.2 g

Protein 6.8 g

16. Creamy Pepper Spread

Preparation Time: 10 minutes
Cooking Time: 15 minutes
Servings: 4

Ingredients:

- 1 lb. red bell peppers chopped and remove seeds
- 1 1/2 tbsp. fresh basil
- 1 tbsp. olive oil
- 1 tbsp. fresh lime juice
- 1 tsp. garlic, minced Pepper
- Salt

Directions:

1. Put all ingredients into the inner pot of the instant pot and stir well.
2. Seal pot with lid and cook on high for 15 minutes.
3. If it is already done, allow to release pressure naturally for 10 minutes, then release remaining using quick release. Remove lid.
4. Transfer bell pepper mixture into the food processor and process until smooth.
5. Serve and enjoy.

Nutrition:
Calories 41 Fat 3.6 g
Carbohydrates 3.5 g
Sugar 1.7 g
Protein 0.4 g

17.   Perfect Queso

Preparation Time: 10 minutes
Cooking Time: 15 minutes
Servings: 16

Ingredients:

- 1 lb. ground beef
- 32 oz. Velveeta cheese, cut into cubes
- 10 oz. can tomato, diced
- 1 1/2 tbsp. taco seasoning
- 1 tsp. chili powder
- One onion, diced Pepper
- Salt

Directions:

1. Set instant pot on sauté mode.
2. Add meat, onion, taco seasoning, chili powder, pepper, and salt into the pot and cook until the heart is no longer pink.
3. Add tomatoes and stir well. Top with cheese and do not mix.
4. Seal pot with lid and cook on high for 4 minutes.
5. Once done, release pressure using quick release. Remove lid.
6. Stir everything well and serve.

Nutrition:
Calories 257 Fat 15.9 g
Carbohydrates 10.2 g Sugar 4.9 g

Protein 21 g

18.   Tasty Spinach Artichoke Dip

Preparation Time: 10 minutes
Cooking Time: 4 minutes
Servings: 10

Ingredients:

- 15 oz. can artichoke hearts, drained
- 1/2 tsp. onion powder
- 1 tsp. garlic, chopped
- 1/2 cup mayonnaise
- 1/2 cup sour cream
- 1/2 cup vegetable broth
- 8 oz. mozzarella cheese, shredded
- 15 oz. parmesan cheese, shredded
- 10 oz. spinach
- 8 oz. cream cheese

Directions:

1. Add all ingredients except parmesan cheese and mozzarella cheese into the instant pot and stir well.
2. Seal pot with lid and cook on high for 4 minutes.
3. Once done, release pressure using quick release. Remove lid.
4. Add parmesan cheese and mozzarella cheese and stir until cheese is melted.
5. Serve and enjoy.

Nutrition:
Calories 372 Fat 27.5 g
Carbohydrates 9.6 g Sugar 1.4 g
Protein 24 g

19.   Yogurt Dip

Preparation time: 10 minutes
Cooking time: 0 minutes
Servings: 6

Ingredients:

- 3 cups Greek yogurt
- 2 tbsp. pistachios, toasted, and chopped
  A pinch of salt and white pepper
- 2 tbsp. mint, chopped
- 1 tbsp. kalamata olives, pitted and chopped
- ¼ cup za'atar spice

- ¼ cup pomegranate seeds
- 1/3 cup olive oil

Directions:

1. In a bowl, combine the yogurt with the pistachios and the rest of the ingredients, whisk well, divide into small cups and serve with pita chips on the side.

Nutrition:

Calories 294

Fat 18g

Fiber 1g

Carbs 21g

Protein 10 g

20. Walnuts Yogurt Dip

Preparation time: 5 minutes

Cooking time: 0 minutes

Servings: 8

Ingredients:

- Three garlic cloves, minced 2 cups Greek yogurt
- ¼ cup dill, chopped
- 1 tbsp. chives, chopped
- ¼ cup walnuts, chopped
- Salt and black pepper to the taste

Directions:

1. In a bowl, mix the garlic with the yogurt and the rest of the ingredients, whisk well, divide into small cups and serve as a party dip.

Nutrition:

Calories 200 Fat 6.5g

Fiber 4.6g

Carbs 15.5g

Protein 8.4 g

21. Cucumber Sandwich Bites

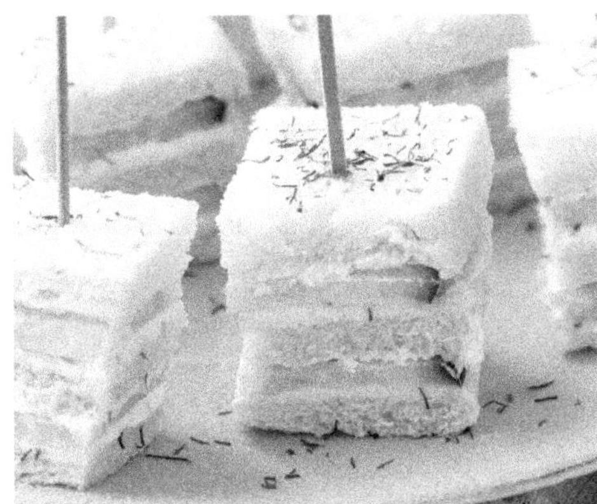

Preparation Time: 5 minutes

Cooking Time: 0 minutes

Servings: 12

Ingredients:

- One cucumber, sliced
- Eight slices of whole wheat bread
- 2 tbsp. cream cheese, soft
- 1 tbsp. chives, chopped
- ¼ cup avocado, peeled, pitted, and mashed
- 1 tsp. mustard
- Salt and black pepper to the taste

Directions:

1. Spread the mashed avocado on each bread slice, also spread the rest of the ingredients except the cucumber slices.
2. Divide the cucumber slices into the bread slices, cut each piece in thirds, arrange on a platter and serve as an appetizer.

Nutrition:

Calories 187 Fat 12.4 g

Fiber 2.1 g Carbs 4.5 g Protein 8.2 g

22. Cucumber Rolls

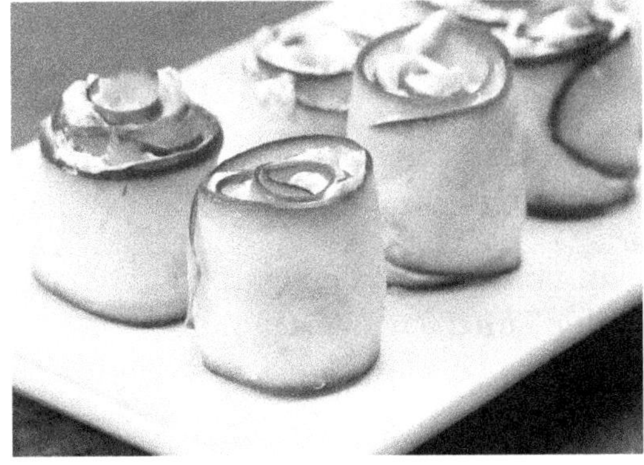

Preparation Time: 5 minutes
Cooking Time: 0 minutes
Servings: 6

Ingredients:

- One big cucumber, sliced lengthwise
- 1 tbsp. parsley, chopped
- 8 ounces canned tuna, drained and mashed
- Salt and black pepper to the taste
- 1 tsp. lime juice

Directions:

1. Arrange cucumber slices on a working surface, divide the rest of the ingredients, and roll.
2. Arrange all the rolls on a platter and serve as an appetizer.

Nutrition:
Calories 200
Fat 6 g
Fiber 3.4 g
Carbs 7.6 g
Protein 3.5 g

23.   Olives and Cheese Stuffed Tomatoes

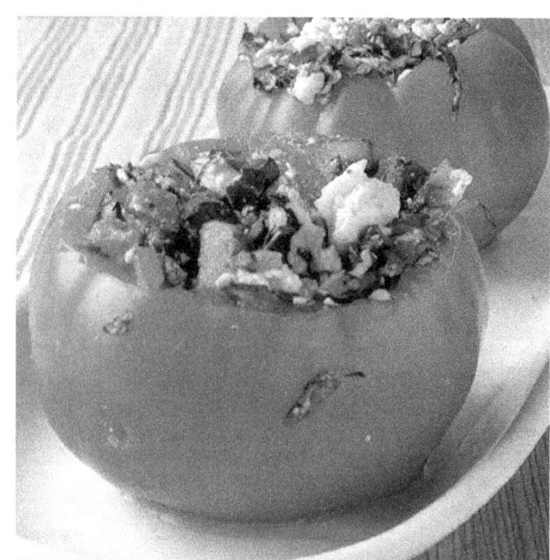

Preparation Time: 10 minutes
Cooking Time: 0 minutes
Servings: 24

Ingredients:

- 24 cherry tomatoes, top cut off, and insides scooped out
- 2 tbsp. olive oil
- ¼ tsp. red pepper flakes
- ½ cup feta cheese, crumbled
- 2 tbsp. black olive paste
- ¼ cup mint, torn

Directions:

1. In a bowl, mix the olives paste with the rest of the ingredients except the cherry tomatoes and whisk.
2. Stuff the cherry tomatoes with this mix, arrange them all on a platter, and serve as an appetizer.

Nutrition:
Calories 136; Fat 8.6 g
Fiber 4.8 g Carbs 5.6 g Protein 5.1 g

24.   Tomato Salsa

Preparation Time: 5 minutes
Cooking Time: 0 minutes
Servings: 6

Ingredients:

- One garlic clove, minced
- 4 tbsp. olive oil
- Five tomatoes, cubed
- 1 tbsp. balsamic vinegar
- ¼ cup basil, chopped
- 1 tbsp. parsley, chopped
- 1 tbsp. chives, chopped
- Salt and black pepper to the taste
- Pita chips for serving

Directions:

1. In a prepared bowl, mix the tomatoes with the garlic and the rest of the ingredients except the pita chips, stir, divide into small cups and serve with the pita chips on the side.

Nutrition:
Calories 160
Fat 13.7 g
Fiber 5.5 g
Carbs 10.1 g
Protein 2.2 g

25. Chili Mango and Watermelon Salsa

Preparation Time: 5 minutes
Cooking Time: 0 minutes
Servings: 12

Ingredients:

- One red tomato, chopped
- Salt and black pepper to the taste
- 1 cup watermelon, seedless, peeled, and cubed
- One red onion, chopped
- Two mangos, peeled and chopped
- Two chili peppers, chopped
- ¼ cup cilantro, chopped
- 3 tbsp. lime juice
- Pita chips for serving

Directions:

1. In a bowl, mix the tomato with the watermelon, the onion, and the rest of the ingredients except the pita chips and toss well.
2. Divide the mix into small cups and serve with pita chips on the side.

Nutrition:
Calories 62 Fat 4g
Fiber 1.3 g
Carbs 3.9 g
Protein 2.3 g

26. Creamy Spinach and Shallots Dip

Preparation Time: 10 minutes
Cooking Time: 0 minutes
Servings: 4

Ingredients:

- 1 pound spinach, roughly chopped
- Two shallots, chopped
- 2 tbsp. mint, chopped
- ¾ cup cream cheese, soft
- Salt and black pepper to the taste

Directions:

1. In your blender, combine the spinach with the shallots and the rest of the ingredients, and pulse well.
2. Divide into small bowls and serve as a party dip.

Nutrition:
Calories 204; Fat 11.5 g
Fiber 3.1 g Carbs 4.2 g
Protein 5.9 g

27. Feta Artichoke Dip

Preparation Time: 10 minutes
Cooking Time: 30 minutes
Servings: 8

Ingredients:

- 8 ounces artichoke hearts, drained and quartered
- ¾ cup basil, chopped
- ¾ cup green olives, pitted and chopped
- 1 cup parmesan cheese, grated
- 5 ounces feta cheese, crumbled

Directions:

1. In your food processor, mix the artichokes with the basil and the rest of the ingredients, pulse well, and transfer to a baking dish.
2. Introduce in the oven, bake at 375° F for 30 minutes and serve as a party dip.

Nutrition:
Calories 186
Fat 12.4 g
Fiber 0.9 g
Carbs 2.6 g
Protein 1.5 g

28. Avocado Dip

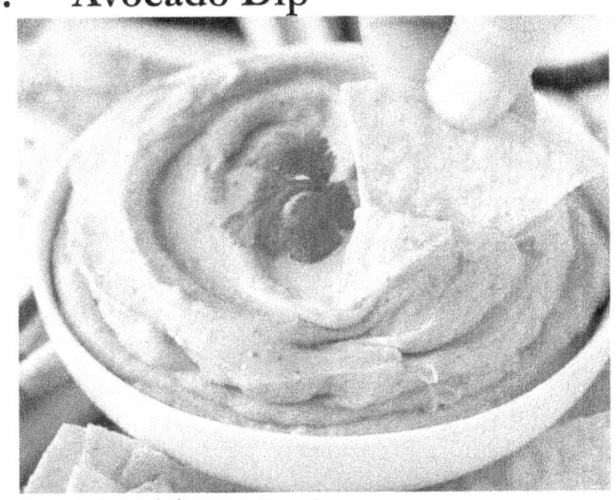

Preparation Time: 5 minutes
Cooking Time: 0 minutes
Servings: 8

Ingredients:

- ½ cup heavy cream
- One green chili pepper, chopped
- Salt and pepper to the taste
- Four avocados, pitted, peeled, and chopped
- 1 cup cilantro, chopped
- ¼ cup lime juice

Directions:

1. In your blender, combine the cream with the avocados and the rest of the ingredients and pulse well.
2. Divide the mix into bowls and serve cold as a party dip.

Nutrition:
Calories 200 Fat 14.5 g
Fiber 3.8 g
Carbs 8.1 g
Protein 7.6 g

29. Goat Cheese and Chives Spread

Preparation Time: 10 minutes
Cooking Time: 0 minute
Servings: 4

Ingredients:

- 2 ounces goat cheese, crumbled
- ¾ cup sour cream
- 2 tbsp. chives, chopped
- 1 tbsp. lemon juice
- Salt and black pepper to the taste
- 2 tbsp. extra virgin olive oil

Directions:

1. In a prepared bowl, mix the goat cheese with the cream and the rest of the ingredients and whisk well.
2. Keep in the fridge for 10 minutes and serve as a party spread.

Nutrition:
Calories 220; Fat 11.5 g;
Fiber 4.8 g; Carbs 8.9 g;
Protein 5.6 g

30. Veggie Fritters

Preparation Time: 10 minutes
Cooking Time: 10 minutes

Servings: 4

Ingredients:

- Two garlic cloves, minced
- Two yellow onions, chopped
- Four scallions, chopped
- Two carrots, grated
- 2 tsp. cumin, ground
- ½ tsp. turmeric powder
- Salt and black pepper to the taste
- ¼ tsp. coriander, ground
- 2 tbsp. parsley, chopped
- ¼ tsp. lemon juice
- ½ cup almond flour
- Two beets, peeled and grated
- Two eggs whisked
- ¼ cup tapioca flour
- 3 tbsp. olive oil

Directions:

1. In a bowl, combine the garlic with the onions, scallions, and the rest of the ingredients except the oil, stir well and shape medium fritters out of this mix.
2. Heat a pan with the oil over medium-high heat, add the fritters, cook for 5 minutes on each side, arrange on a platter and serve.

Nutrition:
Calories 209; Fat 11.2 g;
Fiber 3 g;
Carbs 4.4 g;
Protein 4.8 g

31. White Bean Dip

Preparation Time: 10 minutes
Cooking Time: 0 minute
Servings: 4

Ingredients:

- 15 ounces canned white beans, drained and rinsed
- 6 ounces canned artichoke hearts, drained and quartered
- Four garlic cloves, minced
- 1 tbsp. basil, chopped
- 2 tbsp. olive oil
- Juice of ½ lemon

- Zest of ½ lemon, grated
- Salt and black pepper to the taste

Directions:

1. In your food processor, combine the beans with the artichokes and the rest of the ingredients except the oil and pulse well.
2. Add the oil gradually, pulse the mix again, divide into cups and serve as a party dip.

Nutrition:

Calories 274; Fat 11.7 g;
Fiber 6.5 g; Carbs 18.5 g;
Protein 16.5 g

32.   Eggplant Dip

Preparation Time: 10 minutes
Cooking Time: 40 minutes
Servings: 4

Ingredients:

- One eggplant, poked with a fork
- 2 tbsp. tahini paste
- 2 tbsp. lemon juice
- Two garlic cloves, minced
- 1 tbsp. olive oil
- Salt and black pepper to the taste
- 1 tbsp. parsley, chopped

Directions:

1. Put the eggplant in a roasting pan, bake at 400° F for 40 minutes, cool down, peel and transfer to your food processor.
2. Add the rest of the ingredients except the parsley, pulse well, divide into small bowls and serve as an appetizer with the parsley sprinkled on top.

Nutrition:

Calories 121 Fat 4.3 g
Fiber 1 g Carbs 1.4 g
Protein 4.3 g

33.   Bulgur Lamb Meatballs

Preparation Time: 10 minutes
Cooking Time: 15 minute
Servings: 6

Ingredients:

- One and ½ cups Greek yogurt
- ½ tsp. cumin, ground
- 1 cup cucumber, shredded
- ½ tsp. garlic, minced
- A pinch of salt and black pepper
- 1 cup bulgur
- 2 cups water
- 1-pound lamb, ground
- ¼ cup parsley, chopped
- ¼ cup shallots, chopped
- ½ tsp. allspice, ground
- ½ tsp. cinnamon powder
- 1 tbsp. olive oil

Directions:

1. In a prepared bowl, combine the bulgur with the water, cover the bowl, leave aside for 10 minutes, drain and transfer to a bowl.
2. Add the meat, the yogurt, and the rest of the ingredients except the oil, stir well and shape medium meatballs out of this mix.
3. Heat a pan with the oil over medium-high heat, add the meatballs, cook them for 7 minutes on each side, arrange them all on a platter and serve as an appetizer.

Nutrition:

Calories 300
Fat 9.6 g
Fiber 4.6 g
Carbs 22.6 g
Protein 6.6 g

34.   Cucumber Bites

Preparation Time: 10 minutes
Cooking Time: 0 minutes
Servings: 12

Ingredients:

- 1 English cucumber, sliced into 32 rounds
- 10 ounces hummus
- 16 cherry tomatoes, halved
- 1 tbsp. parsley, chopped
- 1-ounce feta cheese, crumbled

Directions:

1. Spread the hummus on each cucumber round, divide the tomato halves on each, sprinkle the cheese and parsley on to, and serve as an appetizer.

Nutrition:

Calories 162; Fat 3.4 g;
Fiber 2 g; Carbs 6.4 g;
Protein 2.4 g

35. Stuffed Avocado

Preparation Time: 10 minutes
Cooking Time: 0 minute
Servings: 2

Ingredients:

- One avocado halved and pitted
- 10 ounces canned tuna, drained
- 2 tbsp. sun-dried tomatoes, chopped
- One and ½ tbsp. basil pesto
- 2 tbsp. black olives, pitted and chopped
- Salt and black pepper to the taste
- 2 tsp. pine nuts, toasted and chopped
- 1 tbsp. basil, chopped

Directions:

1. In a bowl, combine the tuna with the sun-dried tomatoes and the rest of the ingredients except the avocado and stir.
2. Stuff the avocado halves with the tuna mix and serve as an appetizer.

Nutrition:

Calories 233;
Fat 9 g;
Fiber 3.5 g;
Carbs 11.4 g;
Protein 5.6 g

36. Wrapped Plums

Preparation Time: 5 minutes
Cooking Time: 0 minutes
Servings: 8

Ingredients:

- 2 ounces prosciutto, cut into 16 pieces
- Four plums, quartered
- 1 tbsp. chives, chopped
- A pinch of red pepper flakes, crushed

Directions:

1. Wrap each plum quarter in a prosciutto slice
2. Arrange them all on a platter, sprinkle the chives and pepper flakes all over, and serve.

Nutrition:

Calories 30
Fat 1 g
Fiber 0 g
Carbs 4 g
Protein 2 g

37. Fluffy Bites

Preparation Time: 20 minutes
Cooking Time: 60 minutes
Servings: 12

Ingredients:

- 2 tsp. cinnamon
- 2/3 cup sour cream
- 2 cups heavy cream
- 1 tsp. scraped vanilla bean
- ¼ tsp. cardamom
- Four egg yolks
- Stevia to taste

Directions:

1. Start by whisking your egg yolks until creamy and smooth.
2. Get out a double boiler, and add your eggs with the rest of your ingredients. Mix well.
3. Remove from heat, allowing it to cool until it reaches room temperature.
4. Refrigerate for an hour before whisking well.
5. Pour into molds, and freeze for at least an hour before serving.

Nutrition:

Calories: 363
Protein: 2 g
Fat: 40 g
Carbohydrates: 1 g

38. Coconut Fudge

Preparation Time: 20 minutes
Cooking Time: 60 minutes

Servings: 12

Ingredients:

- 2 cups coconut oil
- ½ cup dark cocoa powder
- ½ cup coconut cream
- ¼ cup almonds, chopped
- ¼ cup coconut, shredded
- 1 tsp. almond extract
- Pinch of salt
- Stevia to taste

Directions:

1. Pour your coconut oil and coconut cream in a bowl, whisking with an electric beater until smooth. Once the mixture becomes smooth and glossy, do not continue.
2. Begin to add in your cocoa powder while mixing slowly, making sure that there aren't any lumps.
3. Add in the rest of your ingredients, and mix well.
4. Line a pan with parchment paper, and freeze until it sets.
5. Slice into squares before serving.

Nutrition:
Calories: 172
Fat: 20 g
Carbohydrates: 3 g

39.   Nutmeg Nougat

Preparation Time: 30 minutes
Cooking Time: 60 minutes
Servings: 12

Ingredients:

- 1 cup heavy cream
- 1 cup cashew butter
- 1 cup coconut, shredded
- ½ tsp. nutmeg
- 1 tsp. vanilla extract, pure
- Stevia to taste

Directions:

1. Melt your cashew butter using a double boiler, and then stir in your vanilla extract, dairy cream, nutmeg, and stevia. Make sure it's mixed well.
2. Remove from heat, allowing it to cool down before refrigerating it for half an hour.
3. Shape into balls, and coat with shredded coconut. Chill for at least two hours then serve.

Nutrition:
Calories: 341
Fat: 34 g
Carbohydrates: 5 g

40.   Sweet Almond Bites

Preparation Time: 30 minutes
Cooking Time: 90 minutes
Servings: 12
Ingredients:

- 18 ounces butter, grass-fed
- 2 ounces heavy cream
- ½ cup Stevia
- 2/3 cup cocoa powder
- 1 tsp. vanilla extract, pure
- 4 tbsp. almond butter

Direction:

1. Use a double boiler and melt your butter before adding in all of your remaining ingredients.
2. Place the mixture into molds, freezing for two hours before serving.

Nutrition:
Calories: 350
Protein: 2 g
Fat: 38 g

CHAPTER 8:

Meat

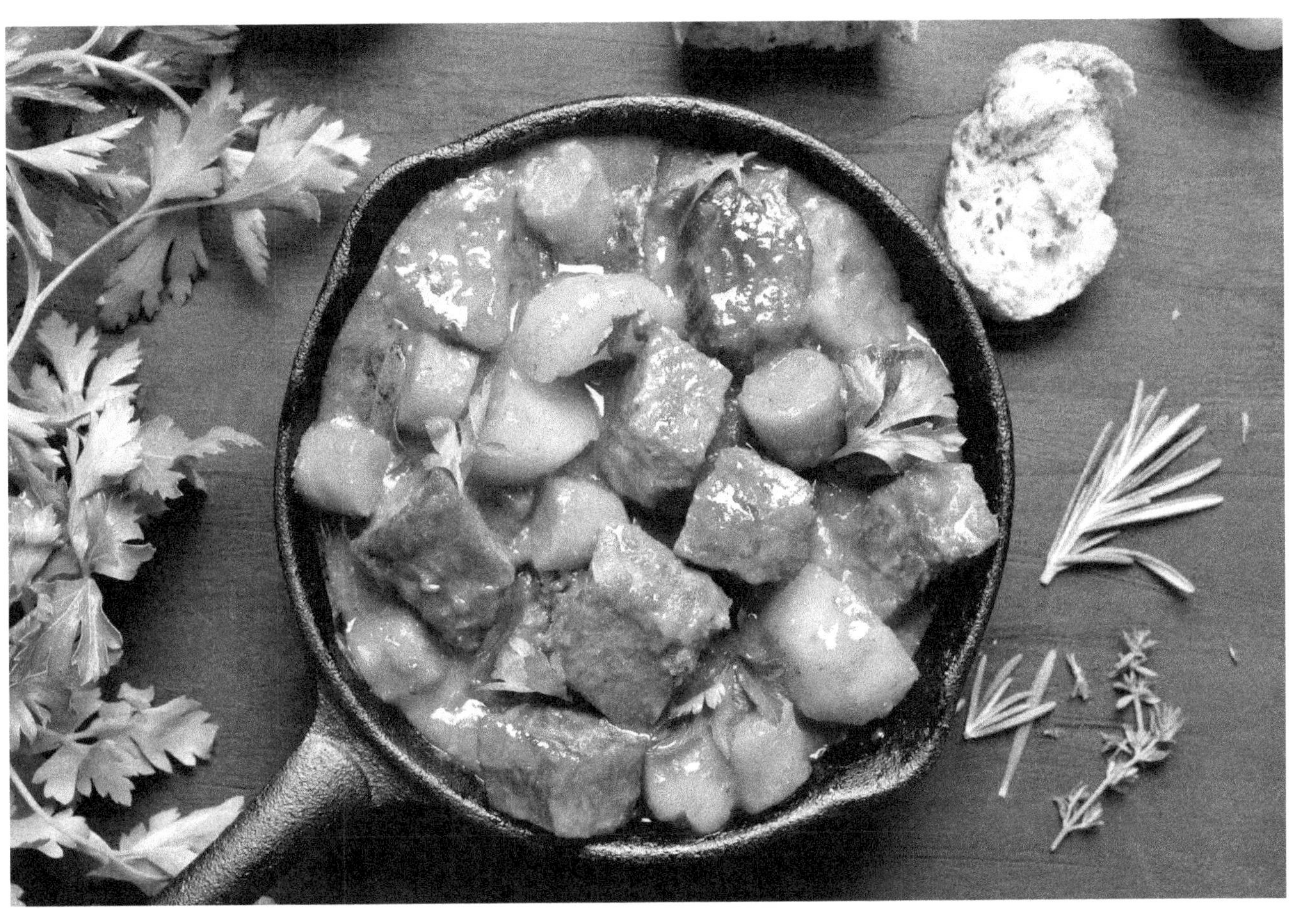

1.   Tasty Beef Stew

Preparation Time: 10 minutes
Cooking Time: 30 minutes
Servings: 4
Ingredients

- 2 1/2 lbs. beef roast, cut into chunks
- 1 cup beef broth
- 1/2 cup balsamic vinegar
- 1 tbsp. honey
- 1/2 tsp. red pepper flakes
- 1 tbsp. garlic, minced
- Pepper Salt

Directions

1. Put all ingredients inside inner pot of the instant pot and stir well.
2. Seal pot with lid and cook on high for 30 minutes.
3. Once done, allow to release pressure naturally. Remove lid. Stir well and serve.

Nutrition:
Calories 562
Fat 18.1 g
Carbohydrates 5.7 g
Protein 87.4 g
Cholesterol 253 mg

2.   Flavorful Beef Bourguignon

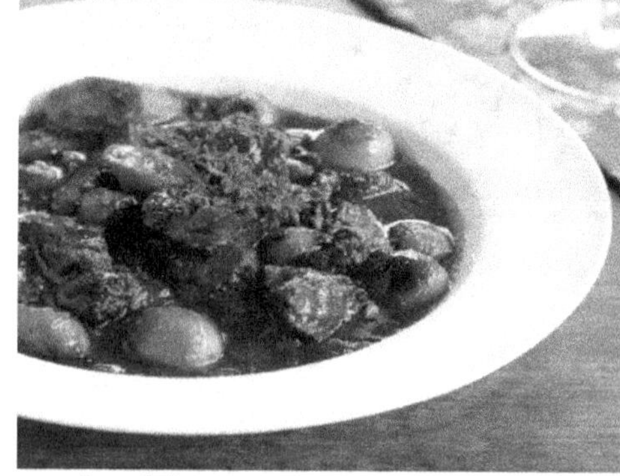

Preparation Time: 10 minutes
Cooking Time: 20 minutes
Servings: 4

Ingredients

- 1 1/2 lbs. beef chuck roast, cut into chunks
- 2/3 cup beef stock
- 2 tbsp. fresh thyme

- One bay leaf
- 1 tsp. garlic, minced
- 8 oz. mushrooms, sliced
- 2 tbsp. tomato paste
- 2/3 cup dry red wine
- One onion, sliced
- Four carrots, cut into chunks
- 1 tbsp. olive oil
- Pepper Salt

Directions

1. Add oil into the instant pot and set the pot on sauté mode. Add meat and sauté until brown. Add onion and sauté until softened.
2. Add remaining ingredients and stir well—seal pot with lid and cook on high for 12 minutes. Once done, allow to release pressure naturally. Remove lid. Stir well and serve.

Nutrition:
Calories 744
Fat 51.3 g
Carbohydrates 14.5 g
Sugar 6.5 g
Protein 48.1 g

3.   Rosemary Creamy Beef

Preparation Time: 10 minutes
Cooking Time: 40 minutes
Servings: 4

Ingredients

- 2 lbs. beef stew meat, cubed
- 2 tbsp. fresh parsley, chopped
- 1 tsp. garlic, minced
- 1/2 tsp. dried rosemary
- 1 tsp. chili powder
- 1 cup beef stock
- 1 cup heavy cream
- One onion, chopped
- 1 tbsp. olive oil
- Pepper Salt

Directions:

Add oil into the instant pot and set the pot on

sauté mode. Add rosemary, garlic, onion, and chili powder and sauté for 5 minutes.

Add meat and cook for 5 minutes. Add remaining ingredients and stir well—seal pot with a lid and cook on high for 30 minutes.

If it is already done, release pressure naturally for 10 minutes, then release remaining using quick release. Remove lid. Serve and enjoy.

Nutrition:

Calories 574 Fat 29 g

Carbohydrates 4.3 g

Protein 70.6 g

Cholesterol 244 mg

4.   Carrot Mushroom Beef Roast

Preparation Time: 10 minutes

Cooking Time: 40 minutes

Servings: 4

Ingredients

- 1 1/2 lbs. beef roast
- 1 tsp. paprika
- 1/4 tsp. dried rosemary
- 1 tsp. garlic, minced
- 1/2 lb. mushrooms sliced
- 1/2 cup chicken stock
- Two carrots, sliced Pepper Salt

Directions

1. Put all ingredients inside the inner pot of the instant pot and stir well. Seal pot with lid and cook on high for 40 minutes.
2. If it is already done, release pressure naturally for 10 minutes, then release remaining using quick release. Remove lid. Slice and serve.

Nutrition:

Calories 345

Fat 10.9 g

Carbohydrates 5.6 g

Protein 53.8 g

Cholesterol 152 mg

5.   Beef with Tomatoes

Preparation Time: 10 minutes

Cooking Time: 40 minutes

Servings: 4

Ingredients:

- 2 lb. beef roast, sliced
- 1 tbsp. chives, chopped
- 1 tsp. garlic, minced
- 1/2 tsp. chili powder
- 2 tbsp. olive oil
- One onion, chopped
- 1 cup beef stock
- 1 tbsp. oregano, chopped
- 1 cup tomatoes, chopped
- Pepper Salt

Directions

1. Add oil into the instant pot and set the pot on sauté mode. Add garlic, onion, and chili powder and sauté for 5 minutes.
2. Add meat and cook for 5 minutes. Add remaining ingredients and stir well—seal pot with lid and cook on high for 30 minutes.
3. When done, release pressure naturally for 10 minutes, then release remaining using quick release. Remove lid. Stir well and serve.

Nutrition:

Calories 511 Fat 21.6 g

Carbohydrates 5.6 g

Sugar 2.5 g

Protein 70.4 g

Cholesterol 203 mg

6.   Beef & Beans

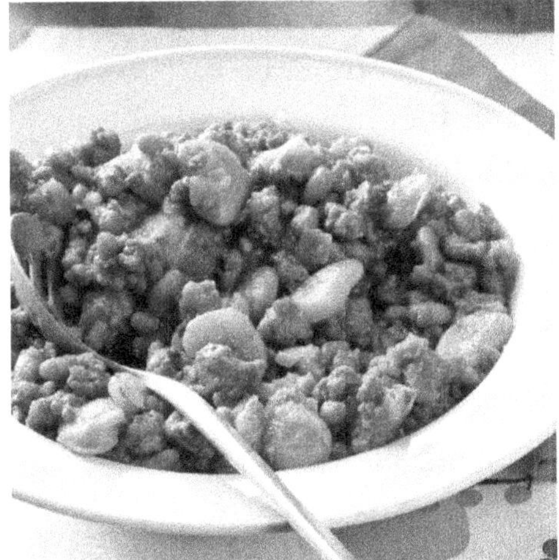

Preparation Time: 10 minutes

Cooking Time: 30 minutes

Servings: 4

Ingredients

- 1 1/2 lbs. beef, cubed
- 8 oz. can tomatoes, chopped
- 8 oz. red beans, soaked overnight, and rinsed
- 1 tsp. garlic, minced
- 1 1/2 cups beef stock
- 1/2 tsp. chili powder
- 1 tbsp. paprika
- 2 tbsp. olive oil, one onion, chopped
- Pepper Salt

Directions

1. Add oil into the instant pot and set the pot on sauté mode. Add meat and cook for 5 minutes. Add garlic and onion and sauté for 5 minutes.
2. Add remaining ingredients and stir well—seal pot with lid and cook on high for 25 minutes. Once done, allow to release pressure naturally. Remove lid. Stir well and serve.

Nutrition:

Calories 604 Fat 18.7 g
Carbohydrates 41.6 g Sugar 4.5 g
Protein 66.6 g
Cholesterol 152 mg

7.   Rosemary Beef Eggplant

Preparation Time: 10 minutes
Cooking Time: 30 minutes
Servings: 4

Ingredients

- 1 lb. beef stew meat, cubed
- 2 tbsp. green onion, chopped
- 1/4 tsp. red pepper flakes
- 1/2 tsp. dried rosemary
- 1/2 tsp. paprika
- 1 cup chicken stock
- One onion, chopped
- One eggplant, cubed
- 2 tbsp. olive oil
- Pepper
- Salt

Directions

1. Add oil into the instant pot and set the pot on sauté mode. Add meat and onion and sauté for 5 minutes. Add remaining ingredients and stir well.
2. Seal pot with lid and cook on high for 25 minutes. Once done, allow to release pressure naturally. Remove lid. Serve and enjoy.

Nutrition:

Calories 315 Fat 14.5 g
Carbohydrates 10 g Protein 36.1 g
Cholesterol 101 mg

8.   Thyme Ginger Garlic Beef

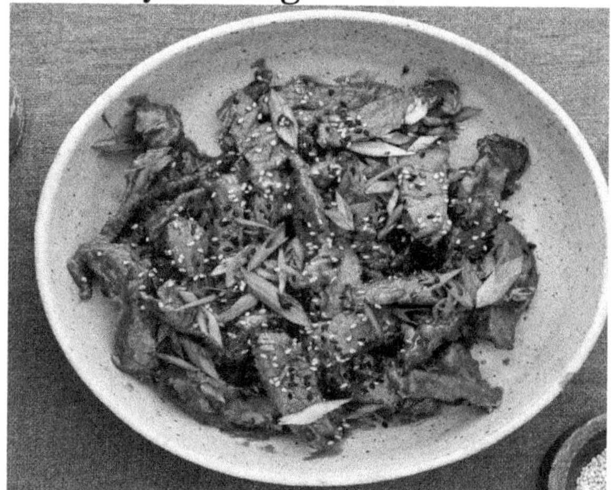

Preparation Time: 10 minutes
Cooking Time: 45 minutes
Servings: 2

Ingredients:

- 1 lb. beef roast
- Two whole cloves
- 1/2 tsp. ginger, grated
- 1/2 cup beef stock
- 1/2 tsp. garlic powder
- 1/2 tsp. thyme
- 1/4 tsp. pepper
- 1/4 tsp. salt

Directions

1. Mix ginger, cloves, thyme, garlic powder, pepper, and salt and rub over beef.
2. Place meat into the instant pot. Pour stock around the meat.

3. Seal pot with lid and cook on high for 45 minutes. Once done, release pressure using quick release.
4. Remove lid. Shred meat using a fork and serve.

Nutrition:

Calories 452 Fat 15.7 g

Carbohydrates 5.2 g Sugar 0.4 g

Protein 70.1 g Cholesterol 203 mg

9.   Garlic & Thyme Pork Chops

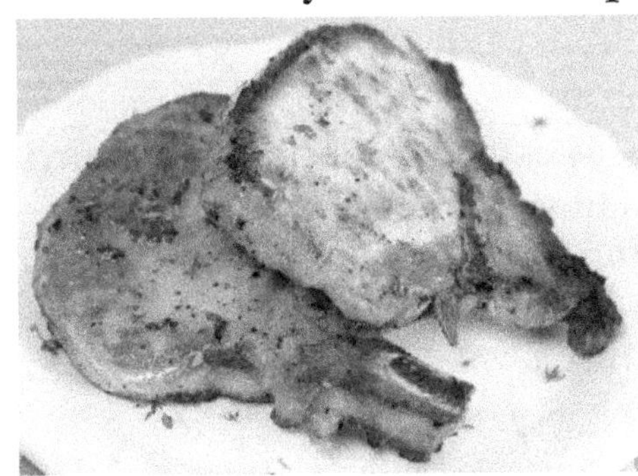

Preparation Time: 10 minutes

Cooking Time: 35 minutes

Servings: 4

Ingredients

- 1 tbsp. olive oil
- Four pork loin chops, boneless
- Salt and black pepper to taste
- Four garlic cloves, minced
- 1 tbsp. thyme, chopped

Directions

1. Preheat the oven to 390 F. Place pork chops, salt, pepper, garlic, thyme, and olive oil in a roasting pan and bake for 10 minutes. Decrease the heat to 360 F and bake for another 25 minutes. Serve with salad.

Nutrition:

Calories 170

Fat 6g

Carbs 2g

Protein 26g

10.   Sweet & Spicy Pork Chops

Preparation Time: 10 minutes

Cooking Time: 20 minutes

Servings: 4

Ingredients

- ½ tsp. cayenne powder
- Four pork chops, boneless
- ¼ cup peach
- 1 tbsp. thyme, chopped
- 2 tbsp. olive oil

Directions:

1. In a bowl, mix peach preserves, olive oil, and cayenne powder.
2. Preheat your grill to medium heat. Rub pork chops with some peach glaze and grill for 10 minutes. Turn the chops, rub more glazes and cook for another 10 minutes. Serve garnished with thyme.

Nutrition:

Calories 240

Fat 12g

Carbs 7g

Protein 24g

11.   Buttermilk Pork Stew

Preparation Time: 10 minutes

Cooking Time: 40 minutes

Servings: 4

Ingredients

- 1 tbsp. avocado oil
- 1 ½ lb. pork meat, boneless and cubed
- One red onion, chopped
- One garlic clove, minced
- ½ cup chicken stock
- 2 tbsp. hot paprika
- Salt and black pepper to taste
- 1 ½ cups buttermilk
- 1 tbsp. cilantro, chopped

Directions

1. Warm the olive oil in a pot over medium heat and sear pork for 5 minutes. Put in onion and garlic and cook for 5 minutes.
2. Stir in stock, paprika, salt, pepper, and buttermilk and bring to a boil; cook for 30 minutes. Top with cilantro to serve.

Nutrition:

Calories 310

Fat 10g

Carbs 16g

Protein 23g

12. Pork Loin with Carrots & Snow Peas

Preparation Time: 10 minutes

Cooking Time: 20 minutes

Servings: 4

Ingredients

- Two carrots, chopped
- Two garlic cloves, minced
- 1 lb. pork loin, boneless and cubed
- 4 oz. snow peas
- 2 tbsp. canola oil
- ¾ cup beef stock
- One onion, chopped Salt, and white pepper to taste

Directions

1. Heat the skillet and put the olive oil over medium heat and sear pork for 5 minutes. Stir in snow peas, carrots, garlic, stock, onion, salt, and pepper and bring to a boil; cook for 15 minutes. Serve right away.

Nutrition:

Calories 340 Fat 18g

Carbs 21g

Protein 28g

13. Chili Lamb Stew

Preparation Time: 10 minutes

Cooking Time: 12 minutes

Servings: 4

Ingredients:

- 1 lb. lamb stew, ground Salt, and black pepper to taste
- 2 tbsp. olive oil
- One onion, chopped 2
- garlic cloves, minced
- 1 tbsp. chili paste
- 2 tbsp. balsamic vinegar
- ¼ cup chicken stock
- ¼ cup mint, chopped

Directions

1. Heat the skillet put the olive oil over medium heat and cook the onion for 3 minutes.
2. Put in lamb stew and cook for another 3 minutes. Stir in salt, pepper, garlic, chili paste, vinegar, stock, and mint and cook for an additional 6 minutes. Serve right away.

Nutrition:

Calories 310

Fat 14g

Carbs 16g

Protein 20g

14. Mustard Pork with Cilantro

Preparation Time: 10 minutes

Cooking Time: 25 minutes

Servings: 4

Ingredients:

- 2 tbsp. olive oil
- One onion, chopped
- 2 lb. pork loin, cut into strips
- ½ cup vegetable stock
- Salt and black pepper to taste
- 2 tsp. mustard
- 1 tbsp. cilantro, chopped

Directions:

1. Heat the skillet put the olive oil over medium heat and cook the onion for 5 minutes.
2. Put in pork loin and cook for another 10 minutes, stirring often. Stir in vegetable stock, salt, pepper, mustard, and cilantro and cook for an additional 10 minutes.

Nutrition:

Calories 300 Fat 13g

Carbs 15g Protein 24g

15. Juicy Pork Chops

Preparation Time: 20 minutes

Cooking Time: 20 minutes

Servings: 4

Ingredients:

- Four pork chops
- ½ cup tomato puree

- Salt and black pepper to taste
- 2 tbsp. olive oil
- 1 tbsp. Italian seasoning
- 1 tbsp. rosemary, chopped

Directions:

1. Preheat the oven to 380 F. Warm olive oil in a skillet over medium heat. Sear pork.
2. Stir in salt, pepper, tomato purée, Italian seasoning, and rosemary and bake for 20 minutes. Serve warm.

Nutrition
Calories: 412 kcal Protein: 41.06 g
Fat: 24.23 g Carbohydrates: 5.21 g

16.   Hot Pork Meatballs

Preparation Time: 10 minutes
Cooking Time: 20 minutes
Servings: 4

Ingredients:

- 1 lb. ground pork
- 3 tbsp. olive oil
- 2 tbsp. parsley, chopped
- Two green onions, chopped
- Four garlic cloves, minced
- One red chili, chopped
- 1 cup veggie stock
- 2 tbsp. hot paprika

Directions:

1. Combine pork, parsley, green onions, garlic, and red chili in a bowl and form medium balls out of the mixture.
2. Heat the skillet put the olive oil, set over medium heat. Sear meatballs for 8 minutes on all sides. Stir in stock and hot paprika and simmer for another 12 minutes. Serve warm.

Nutrition:
Calories 240
Fat 19g
Carbs 12g
Protein 15g

17.   Orange Lamb with Dates

Preparation Time: 30 minutes
Cooking Time: 30 minutes

Servings: 4

Ingredients:

- 2 tbsp. olive oil
- 1 tbsp. dates, chopped
- 1 lb. lamb, cubed
- One garlic clove, minced
- One onion, grated
- 2 tbsp. orange juice
- Salt and black pepper to taste
- 1 cup vegetable stock

Directions:

1. Heat the skillet put the olive oil, set over medium heat and cook onion and garlic for 5 minutes. Put in lamb and cook for another 5 minutes.
2. Stir in dates, orange juice, salt, pepper, and stock and bring to a boil; cook for 20 minutes. Serve right away.

Nutrition:
Calories 298 Fat 14g
Carbs 19g
Protein 17g

18.   Dill Beef Brisket

Preparation Time: 10 minutes
Cooking Time: 50 minutes
Servings: 4

Ingredients:

- 2 1/2 lbs. beef brisket, cut into cubes
- 2 1/2 cups beef stock
- 2 tbsp. dill, chopped
- One celery stalk, chopped
- One onion, sliced
- 1 tbsp. garlic, minced
- Pepper Salt

Directions:

1. Put all ingredients into the inner pot of the instant pot and stir well. Seal pot with lid and cook on high for 50 minutes.
2. When done, release pressure naturally for 10 minutes, then release remaining using quick release. Remove lid. Serve and enjoy.

Nutrition:
Calories 556

Fat 18.1 g
Carbohydrates 4.3 g
Sugar 1.3 g
Protein 88.5 g
Cholesterol 253 mg

19.   Meatloaf

Preparation Time: 10 minutes
Cooking Time: 35 minutes
Servings: 6
Ingredients:

- 2 lbs. ground beef
- Two eggs, lightly beaten
- 1/4 tsp. dried basil
- 3 tbsp. olive oil
- 1/2 tsp. dried sage
- 1 1/2 tsp. dried parsley
- 1 tsp. oregano
- 2 tsp. thyme
- 1 tsp. rosemary
- Pepper and Salt

Directions:

1. Pour 1 1/2 cups of water into the instant pot, then place the trivet in the pot.
2. Spray loaf pan with cooking spray. Add all ingredients into the mixing bowl and mix until well combined.
3. Transfer meat mixture into the prepared loaf pan and place loaf pan on top of the pot's trivet. Seal pot with lid and cook on high for 35 minutes.
4. When done, allow to release pressure naturally for 10 minutes, then release remaining using quick release. Remove lid. Serve and enjoy.

Nutrition:
Calories 365
Fat 18 g
Carbohydrates 0.7 g
Protein 47.8 g
Cholesterol 190 mg

20.   Spicy Beef Chili Verde

Preparation Time: 10 minutes
Cooking Time: 23 minutes
Servings: 2

Ingredients:

- 1/2 lb. beef stew meat, cut into cubes
- 1/4 tsp. chili powder
- 1 tbsp. olive oil
- 1 cup chicken broth
- 1 Serrano pepper, chopped
- 1 tsp. garlic, minced
- One small onion, chopped
- 1/4 cup grape tomatoes, chopped
- 1/4 cup tomatillos, chopped
- Pepper Salt

Directions:

1. Add oil into the instant pot and set the pot on sauté mode. Add garlic and onion and sauté for 3 minutes.
2. Add remaining ingredients and stir well—seal pot with a lid and cook on high for 20 minutes. Once done, allow to release pressure naturally. Remove lid. Stir well and serve.

Nutrition:
Calories 317
Fat 15.1 g
Carbohydrates 6.4 g
Sugar 2.6 g
Protein 37.8 g
Cholesterol 101 mg

21.   Moroccan Beef Koftas

Preparation Time: 5 minutes
Cooking Time: 13 minutes
Servings: 2

Ingredients:

- 1/2 pound ground beef
- One small red onion, finely chopped
- 1 tsp. garlic, minced
- 1 tbsp. olive oil
- Sea salt to taste
- Ground black pepper, to taste
- 1/4 tsp. ground coriander
- 1/2 tsp. paprika
- 1/2 tsp. turmeric

- 1/4 tsp. ground cumin
- 1/4 tsp. allspice

Directions

1. Combine thoroughly all ingredients in a mixing bowl.
2. Shape the meat into two thick sausages and thread a bamboo skewer through each sausage.
3. Preheat your grill for medium-high heat. Lower the koftas onto a lightly oiled grill. Grill for about 13 minutes, turning them over once or twice to promote even cooking.
4. An instant-read thermometer should read160 degrees F. Serve with lemon slices or cold plain yogurt if desired. Bon appétit!

Nutrition:
Calories: 308 Fat: 21.4g
Carbs: 6.9g Protein: 23.1g

22.   Beef Tenderloin Salad

Preparation Time: 10 minutes
Cooking Time: 10 minutes
Servings: 4

Ingredients

- 2 tbsp. olive oil
- 1 pound beef tenderloin, sliced
- Sea salt to taste
- Ground black pepper, to taste
- 1/2 tsp. paprika
- 1 tsp. oregano
- One red onion, sliced
- 2 Roma tomatoes, sliced
- 1 Persian cucumber, sliced
- 2 cups Romaine lettuce, torn into pieces
- 2 tbsp. red wine vinegar
- One avocado, peeled and sliced
- 4 ounces canned cannellini beans, drained
- 1 (6 ½-inch) pita, cut into wedges and toasted

Directions

1. Pat dries the beef tenderloin with paper towels. Season the meat with salt, black pepper, paprika, and oregano.
2. Then, cook the steaks on the preheated grill, turning them over once or twice. Cook for about 10 minutes or until slightly charred.
3. Cut the beef into strips and then place them in a salad bowl. Add in the remaining ingredients, except for the pita; toss to combine well.
4. Top your salad with the toasted pita and serve. Bon appétit!

Nutrition:
Calories: 485 Fat: 39.3g
Carbs: 13g Protein: 23.3g

23.   Herb and Wine Beef Stew

Preparation Time: 5 minutes
Cooking Time: 55 minutes
Servings: 4

Ingredients

- 2 tbsp. olive oil
- Sea salt
- Freshly ground black pepper, to taste
- 1 tsp. smoked paprika
- 2 pounds beef stew meat, boneless and cut into bite-sized cubes
- One red onion, chopped
- 1 pound Yukon Gold potatoes, peeled and diced
- Two carrots, sliced
- Three cloves garlic, minced
- Two tomatoes, pureed
- 2 cups beef bone broth
- 1/2 cup dry red wine
- Two bay leaves
- Two thyme sprigs
- Two rosemary sprigs

Directions

1. Heat the olive oil in a heavy-bottomed pot over a medium-high flame. Once hot, sear the meat for about 4 minutes until no longer pink; reserve.

2. Season the meat with salt, black pepper, and smoked paprika.

3. Add in the vegetables and continue sautéing for about 5 minutes or until they are crisp-tender.

4. Put the meat back to the pot along with the pureed tomatoes, beef bone broth, red wine, bay leaves, thyme, and rosemary. Bring to a boil and immediately reduce the heat to a simmer.

5. Let it simmer, partially covered, for about 50 minutes or until everything is cooked through.

6. Ladle into individual bowls. Bon appétit!

Nutrition:
Calories: 481 Fat: 16.8g
Carbs: 27.1g
Protein: 55.4g

24. Classic Italian Stir-Fry

Preparation Time: 5 minutes
Cooking Time: 11 minutes
Servings: 3

Ingredients

- 2 tbsp. olive oil
- 3/4 pound beef brisket, cut into bite-sized strips
- 2 Italian peppers, sliced
- 1 cup cauliflower florets
- One red onion, sliced
- 1 cup brown Italian mushrooms, sliced
- One medium zucchini, julienned
- Two garlic cloves, sliced
- 1/2 tsp. dried basil
- 1 tsp. dried oregano
- 1/2 tsp. crushed red pepper flakes
- Salt and ground black pepper, to taste
- 1/2 cup Greek olives, pitted and sliced

Directions

1. In a prepared large skillet, heat the olive oil until sizzling. Then, stir-fry the beef for about 5 minutes until no longer pink. Place the meat to one side of the skillet.

2. Add in the peppers, cauliflower, and onion and continue to cook for 3 minutes more.

3. Now, stir in the mushrooms, zucchini, garlic, basil, oregano, red pepper flakes, salt, and black pepper; stir-fry for a further 3 minutes or until the vegetables are just tender and fragrant.

4. Top with the olives and serve warm. Bon appétit!

Nutrition:
Calories: 369 Fat: 28.5g
Carbs: 10.1g Protein: 19.4g

25. Beef Salad with Green Beans

Preparation Time: 10 minutes
Cooking Time: 10 minutes
Servings: 4

Ingredients

- 3/4 pound beef tenderloin, fat trimmed, sliced
- Sea salt to taste
- Ground black pepper, to taste
- 1/2 tsp. red pepper flakes, crushed
- 1 tbsp. olive oil
- 1/2 tsp. dried oregano
- 1/2 tsp. dried rosemary
- 1/2 pound green beans
- One red onion, sliced
- One garlic clove, minced
- 1 Persian cucumber, sliced
- One tomato, sliced
- Two roasted peppers, deseeded and sliced
- One green bell pepper, sliced
- 2 tbsp. fresh parsley, roughly chopped
- 2 tbsp. fresh basil, roughly chopped
- 2 tbsp. fresh mint leaves, roughly chopped
- 1 tbsp. lemon juice
- 4 tbsp. extra-virgin olive oil
- 2 cups butterhead lettuce
- 2 cups baby spinach

Directions

1. Place the green bean in a saucepan and cover it with cold water (2 inches above

them). Bring to a boil and turn the heat to a simmer.

2. Let it simmer for about 5 minutes or until they are crisp-tender; drain the green bean; place them in a bowl of the ice water; drain and reserve.

3. Sprinkle the salt, black pepper, and red pepper evenly over the steaks. Heat the olive oil in a cast-iron skillet over a high flame.

4. Once hot, cook the stakes for 3 to 4 minutes per side or until browned. Reduce the heat to medium-low; add in the oregano and rosemary and continue to sauté an additional 30 seconds or until fragrant.

5. Cut the steaks into strips and transfer them to a salad bowl. Add in the remaining ingredients and toss to coat.

6. Top with the green beans. Bon appétit!

Nutrition:
Calories: 434
Fat: 35.3g
Carbs: 10.5g
Protein: 18.4g

26. Beef and Vegetable Skillet with Cheese

Preparation Time: 10 minutes
Cooking Time: 15 minutes
Servings: 4

Ingredients

- 2 tbsp. olive oil
- 1 pound flank steak, sliced
- One red onion, sliced
- One red bell pepper, sliced
- One zucchini, sliced
- Two cloves garlic, minced
- Sea salt to taste
- Ground black pepper, to taste
- 1 tsp. dried oregano
- 1 tsp. dried basil
- 1 tsp. dried rosemary
- 1/2 cup chicken bone broth
- 2 ounces parmesan cheese, grated

Directions

1. In a prepared large skillet, heat the olive oil until sizzling. Then, stir-fry the beef for about 5 minutes until no longer pink. Place the meat to one side of the skillet.

2. Add in the onion and peppers, and continue to cook for 3 minutes more.

3. Now, stir in the zucchini, garlic, salt, black pepper, basil, oregano, rosemary, and chicken bone broth; stir-fry for a further 3 minutes or until the vegetables are just tender and fragrant.

4. Top with the cheese and remove from the heat; allow it to sit, covered, for about 5 minutes until the cheese has melted. Bon appétit!

Nutrition:
Calories: 335 Fat: 18.5g
Carbs: 5.5g
Protein: 35.4g

27. Chunky Beef and Cannellini Bean Casserole

Preparation Time: 5 minutes
Cooking Time: 35 minutes
Servings: 4

Ingredients

- 2 tbsp. olive oil
- One ¼ pounds ground chuck
- One red onion, chopped
- Two garlic cloves, minced
- 1 Italian pepper, deseeded and sliced
- 8 ounces canned cannellini beans, rinsed
- 1 cup marinara sauce
- 1 cup chicken bone broth
- 3 ounces tortilla chips, crushed
- 1 cup parmesan cheese, grated

Directions

1. Heat the olive oil in a frying pan over medium-high heat. Now, brown the ground chuck until it is no longer pink or about 5 minutes; crumble it with a fork.

2. Add in the onion, garlic, and peppers, and continue cooking for 2 minutes longer.

3. Transfer the cooked meat mixture to a lightly oiled casserole dish. Now, stir in

the beans, marinara sauce, and chicken bone broth.

4. Top with the crushed tortilla chips and parmesan cheese.

5. Bake in the preheated oven at 350 degrees F for 30 minutes or until the cheese is hot and bubbly. Bon appétit!

Nutrition:
Calories: 675 Fat: 34.1g
Carbs: 38g Protein: 54.4g

28. Beef and Mushroom Mélange

Preparation Time: 5 minutes
Cooking Time: 40 minutes
Servings: 4

Ingredients

- 2 tbsp. olive oil
- 1 ½ pounds lean chuck steak, cut into bite-sized chunks
- Sea salt to taste
- Ground black pepper, to taste
- 1 tsp. hot paprika
- One red onion, chopped
- One red pepper, deseeded and sliced
- 3/4 pound brown Cremini mushrooms, sliced
- Three cloves garlic, minced
- 2 cups roasted vegetable broth
- 1 cup cream of mushroom soup
- 1/2 cup dry red wine
- 1/2 pound penne pasta
- 1/4 cup scallions, roughly chopped

Directions

1. Heat the olive oil in a heavy-bottomed pot over medium-high flame. Once hot, sear the beef for about 6 minutes, until no longer pink. Season the meat with salt, black pepper, and paprika and reserve.

2. Add in the vegetables and continue sautéing for about 5 minutes or until they are crisp-tender. Put in the garlic and continue to sauté an additional 30 seconds until aromatic.

3. Add the meat back to the pot along with the broth, mushroom soup, wine, and penne pasta. Bring to a rolling boil and immediately turn the heat to a simmer.

4. Let it simmer, partially covered, for about 30 minutes or until everything is cooked through.

5. Ladle into individual bowls, garnish with freshly chopped scallions, and serve hot. Bon appétit!

Nutrition:
Calories: 605
Fat: 22.5g Carbs: 59.5g
Protein: 44.4g

29. Grilled Steak Salad with Cheese

Preparation Time: 10 minutes
Cooking Time: 10 minutes
Servings: 4

Ingredients

- 3/4 pound beef flank steak, sliced
- Sea salt to taste
- Ground black pepper, to taste
- 1/2 tsp. cayenne pepper
- 2 tbsp. olive oil
- 1/4 cup radishes, thinly sliced
- 1/2 cup scallions, sliced
- One medium tomato, sliced
- 2 tbsp. extra-virgin olive oil
- 1/4 cup balsamic vinegar
- 1 tsp. Greek seasoning mix
- 2 cups baby spinach
- 1/3 cup black olives, pitted and sliced
- 1/2 cup feta cheese, crumbled

Directions

1. Pat dries the beef tenderloin with paper towels. Season the meat with salt, black pepper, and cayenne pepper.

2. Drizzle the steaks with olive oil.

3. Then, cook the steaks on the preheated grill, turning them periodically to promote even cooking. Cook until slightly charred or for about 10 minutes.

4. Cut the beef into strips and then place them in a salad bowl. Add in the

remaining ingredients, except for the cheese; toss to combine well.

5. Top your salad with the crumbled feta cheese and serve at room temperature. Bon appétit!

Nutrition:
Calories: 330
Fat: 23.3g
Carbs: 7.4g
Protein: 22g

30. Beef with Portobello Mushrooms and Cheese

Preparation Time: 5 minutes
Cooking Time: 20 minutes
Servings: 4

Ingredients

- 2 tbsp. olive oil
- 1 pound chuck roast, cut into bite-sized pieces
- One medium leek, sliced
- One carrot, julienned
- One small-sized eggplant, peeled and sliced
- 1 cup Portobello mushrooms, sliced
- Two garlic cloves, sliced
- Seas salt and ground black pepper, to taste
- 1 tbsp. Greek seasoning mix
- 2 tbsp. dry red wine
- 1/2 cup Pecorino Romano cheese, grated

Directions

1. In a large skillet, heat the olive oil until sizzling. Then, cook the beef for about 5 minutes until no longer pink. Place the meat to one side of the skillet.
2. Add in the leek, carrot, and eggplant, and continue to cook for 3 minutes more.
3. Now, stir in the mushrooms, garlic, salt, black pepper, and Greek seasoning mix; cook for a further 3 minutes or until the vegetables are crisp-tender, adding the wine periodically.
4. Top with the cheese, cover, and allow it to melt for 4 to 5 minutes. Bon appétit!

Nutrition:
Calories: 328
Fat: 16.9g
Carbs: 15.9g
Protein: 29.5g

31. Ground Beef, Vegetable and Cheese Bake

Preparation Time: 10 minutes
Cooking Time: 40 minutes
Servings: 4

Ingredients

- 1 tbsp. olive oil
- One ¼ pounds ground beef
- One red onion, chopped
- Two garlic cloves, minced
- One eggplant, peeled and diced
- 8 ounces canned red kidney beans, drained and rinsed
- 1 cup tomato puree
- 1 cup cream of mushroom soup
- 1 cup breadcrumbs
- 1 cup Pecorino-Romano cheese, shredded

Directions

1. Heat the olive oil in a frying pan over medium-high heat. Once hot, brown the ground beef for about 5 minutes, crumbling it with a fork.
2. Add in the onion, garlic, and eggplant, and continue to cook for 2 minutes longer or until they are crisp-tender.
3. Transfer the cooked meat mixture to a lightly oiled casserole dish. Now, stir in the beans, tomato puree, and soup.
4. Top with the breadcrumbs and shredded cheese.
5. Bake your casserole in the preheated oven at 350 degrees F for 30 minutes or until the cheese has melted. Bon appétit!

Nutrition:
Calories: 588
Fat: 29g
Carbs: 37.4g
Protein: 44.5g

## 32.	Chunky Hamburger Soup with Green Beans

Preparation Time: 5 minutes
Cooking Time: 25 minutes
Servings: 4

Ingredients

- 1 tbsp. olive oil
- 3/4 pound ground chuck
- One red onion, diced
- Two carrots, chopped
- One celery stalk, chopped
- One red bell pepper, chopped
- 1 tsp. ginger-garlic paste
- 4 cups beef bone broth
- One ripe tomato, pureed
- 1 tsp. Italian seasoning mix
- Two bay leaves
- Sea salt to taste
- Ground black pepper, to taste
- 1 cup green beans, trimmed

Directions

1. Heat the olive oil in a heavy-bottomed pot over medium-high heat. Once hot, brown the ground beef for about 4 minutes, crumbling with a fork.
2. Now, stir in the vegetables and continue to sauté for 3 to 4 minutes or until crisp-tender.
3. Add in the ginger-garlic paste, broth, tomato, and seasonings, bringing to a boil. Let it simmer, covered, for 10 to 15 minutes or until cooked through.
4. Stir in the green beans and continue to simmer for 5 minutes more until crisp-tender.
5. Ladle into individual bowls and serve hot. Bon appétit!

Nutrition:
Calories: 254
Fat: 11.7g
Carbs: 12.1g
Protein: 23.4g

## 33.	Classic Greek-Style Meatballs

Preparation Time: 10 minutes
Cooking Time: 6 minutes
Servings: 5

Ingredients

Meatballs:

- 1 ½ pound ground chuck
- One red onion, chopped
- Two garlic cloves, pressed
- One bell pepper, chopped
- One pepperoncino, minced
- Sea salt to taste
- Ground black pepper, to taste
- 1/2 tsp. dried oregano
- 1/2 tsp. dried basil
- 1/2 tsp. dried rosemary
- 1 tsp. dried parsley flakes
- One egg
- 1/2 cup seasoned breadcrumbs

Tzatziki Sauce:

- 1/2 cup Greek-style yogurt
- 1/2 cucumber, minced
- 1/2 tsp. dried dill
- Two cloves garlic, pressed
- Sea salt to taste
- Ground black pepper, to taste

Directions

1. Thoroughly combine the ingredients for the meatballs, mix well, and shape the mixture into small balls.
2. Preheat a large frying pan over medium-high heat; sear the meatballs for 5 to 6 minutes until nicely browned.
3. Then, make the tzatziki sauce by whisking the ingredients. Serve the meatballs with the sauce on the side. Enjoy!

Nutrition:
Calories: 305
Fat: 12.7g
Carbs: 14g
Protein: 31.4g

## 34.	Beef Salad Niçoise

Preparation Time: 10 minutes
Cooking Time: 25 minutes
Servings: 4

Ingredients

- Two small red potatoes
- Two large eggs
- 1 pound flank steak, sliced
- Sea salt, to taste
- Freshly ground black pepper, to taste
- 1/2 cup scallions, sliced
- 1/2 cup radishes, thinly sliced
- 1 Greek cucumber, sliced
- 1 Italian pepper, sliced
- 1 cup grape tomatoes, halved
- 4 tbsp. extra-virgin olive oil, divided
- 1 tbsp. champagne vinegar
- 1 tsp. Dijon mustard
- 2 cups Romaine lettuce, torn into pieces
- 16 niçoise olives

Directions

1. Place the potatoes and eggs in a large saucepan; cover with cold water (2 inches above them). Bring to a boil; immediately, reduce heat to medium-low, and cook for 6 to 8 minutes.
2. Transfer the eggs to an ice water-filled bowl. Peel the eggs and cut them into slices; reserve.
3. Continue to boil potatoes for a further 12 to 14 minutes or until fork-tender. Let them cool before cutting into thick slices; reserve.
4. Season the meat with salt and black pepper.
5. Then, cook the steaks on the preheated grill, turning them periodically to promote even cooking. Cook for about 10 minutes until slightly charred.
6. Cut the beef into strips and place them in a salad bowl. Add in the remaining ingredients and toss to combine well.
7. Top your salad with hard-boiled eggs and potatoes. Bon appétit!

Nutrition:
Calories: 412
Fat: 24.7g
Carbs: 18.4g
Protein: 30.2g

35. Ground Beef Soup with Sweet Corn

Preparation Time: 10 minutes
Cooking Time: 40 minutes
Servings: 3

Ingredients

- 1 tbsp. olive oil
- 1/2 pound ground chuck
- Two carrots, sliced
- 1 Italian pepper, sliced
- Two sweet potatoes, sliced
- One medium leek, chopped
- One parsnip, sliced
- One ripe tomato, pureed
- 2 ½ cups beef bone broth
- Sea salt and ground black pepper, to taste
- 1 tsp. poultry seasoning mix
- 1/2 tsp. dried oregano
- 1/2 tsp. dried basil
- 1/2 tsp. dried rosemary
- 1 cup sweet corn kernels

Directions

1. Heat the olive oil in a heavy-bottomed pot over medium-high heat. Once hot, brown the ground chuck for about 4 minutes, crumbling with a fork.
2. Now, stir in the vegetables and continue to sauté for 3 to 4 minutes or until crisp-tender.
3. Add in the tomato, beef bone broth, and seasonings, bringing to a boil. Let it simmer, covered, for 25 minutes or until cooked through.
4. Stir in the corn kernels and continue to simmer for 5 minutes more until warmed through.
5. Ladle into individual bowls and serve hot. Bon appétit!

Nutrition:
Calories: 339
Fat: 11.5g
Carbs: 43g
Protein: 19.5g

CHAPTER 9:

Vegetable

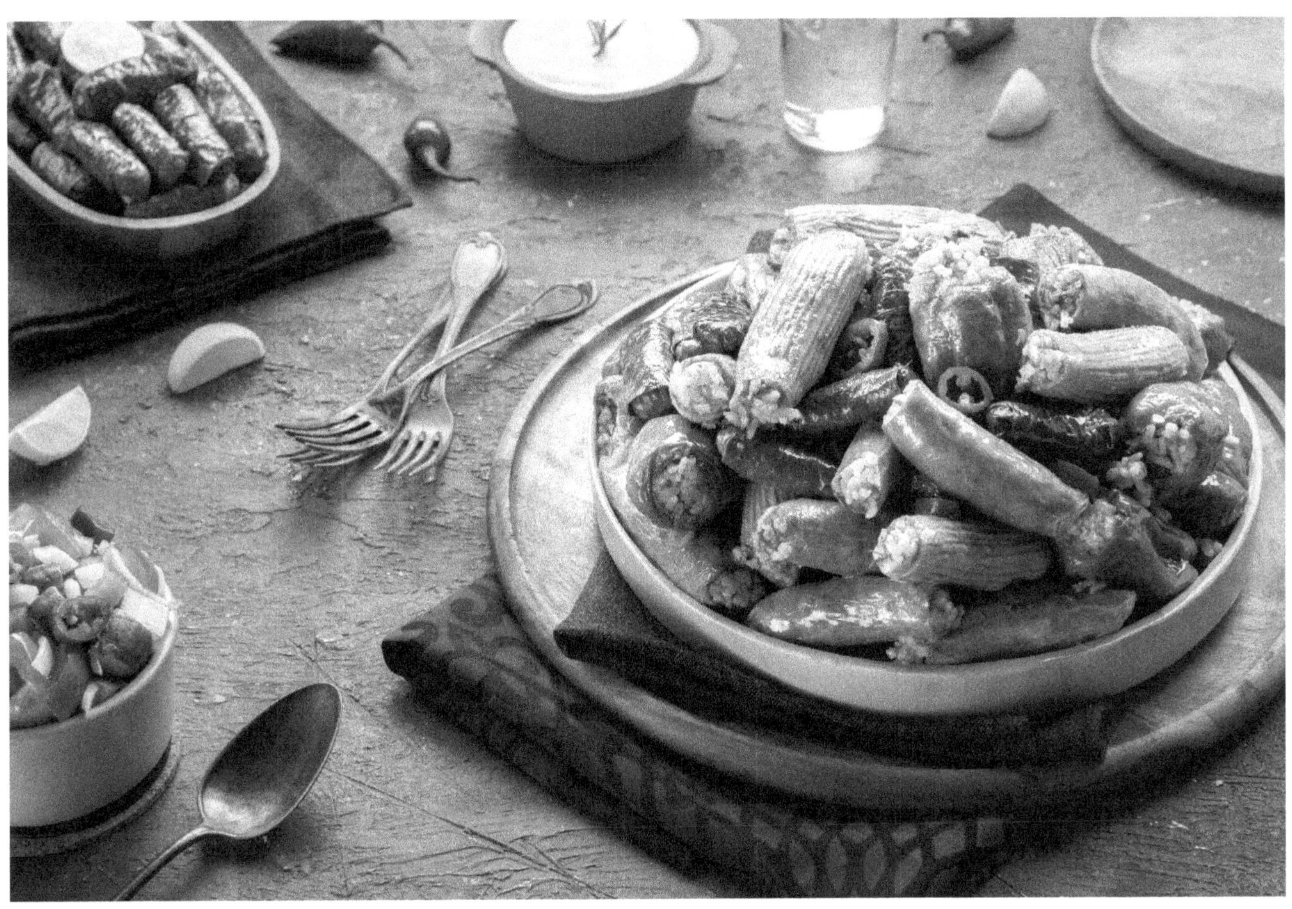

1.   Potato Salad

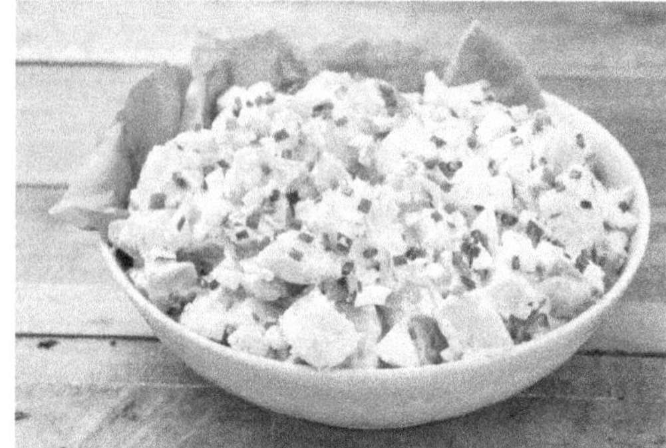

Preparation Time: 10 minutes
Cooking Time: 10 minutes
Servings: 8

Ingredients:

- 5 cups potato, cubed
- 1/4 cup fresh parsley, chopped
- 1/4 tsp. red pepper flakes
- 1 tbsp. olive oil
- 1/3 cup mayonnaise
- 1/2 tbsp. oregano
- 2 tbsp. capers
- 3/4 cup feta cheese, crumbled
- 1 cup olives, halved
- 3 cups of water
- 3/4 cup onion, chopped
- Pepper
- Salt

Directions:

1. Add potatoes, onion, and salt into the instant pot.
2. Seal pot with lid and cook on high for 3 minutes.
3. Once done, release pressure using quick release. Remove lid.
4. Remove potatoes from the pot and place in a large mixing bowl.
5. Add remaining ingredients and stir everything well.
6. Serve and enjoy.

Nutrition:
Calories 152 Fat 9.9 g
Carbohydrates 13.6 g
Sugar 2.1 g
Protein 3.5 g
Cholesterol 15 mg

2.   Greek Green Beans

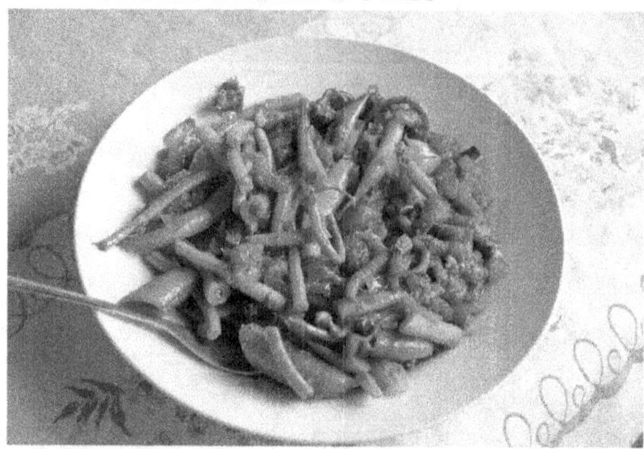

Preparation Time: 10 minutes
Cooking Time: 15 minutes
Servings: 4

Ingredients:

- 1 lb. green beans, remove stems
- Two potatoes, quartered
- 1 1/2 onion, sliced
- 1 tsp. dried oregano
- 1/4 cup dill, chopped
- 1/4 cup fresh parsley, chopped
- One zucchini, quartered
- 1/2 cup olive oil
- 1 cup of water
- k14.5 oz. can tomatoes, diced
- Pepper
- Salt

Directions

1. Add all ingredients into the inner pot of the instant pot and stir everything well.
2. Seal pot with lid and cook on high for 15 minutes.
3. Once done, release pressure using quick release. Remove lid.
4. Stir well and serve.

Nutrition:
Calories 381
Fat 25.8 g
Carbohydrates 37.7 g
Sugar 9 g
Protein 6.6 g

3. Healthy Vegetable Medley

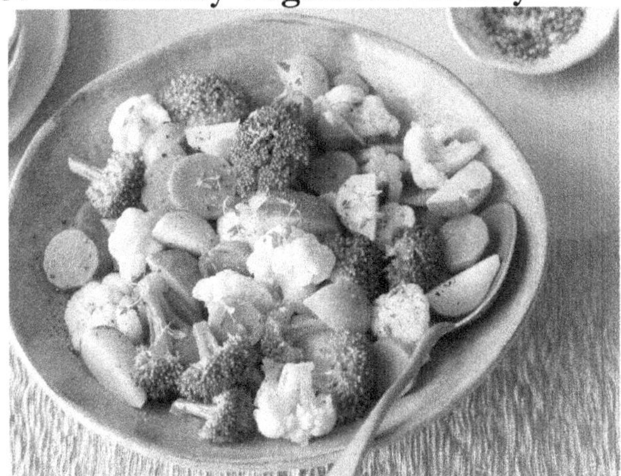

Preparation Time: 10 minutes
Cooking Time: 17 minutes
Servings: 6

Ingredients

- 3 cups broccoli florets
- One sweet potato, chopped
- 1 tsp. garlic, minced
- 14 Oz coconut milk
- 28 Oz can get tomatoes, chopped
- 14 oz. can chickpeas, drained and rinsed
- One onion, chopped
- 1 tbsp. olive oil
- 1 tsp. Italian seasoning
- Pepper
- Salt

Directions

1. Add oil into the inner pot of the instant pot and set the pot on sauté mode.
2. Add garlic and onion and sauté until onion is softened.
3. Add remaining ingredients and stir everything well.
4. Seal pot with lid and cook on high for 12 minutes.
5. Once done, allow to release pressure naturally for 10 minutes, then release remaining using quick release. Remove lid.
6. Stir well and serve.

Nutrition:
Calories 322 Fat 19.3 g
Carbohydrates 34.3 g Sugar 9.6 g
Protein 7.9 g Cholesterol 1 mg

4. Spicy Zucchini

Preparation Time: 10 minutes
Cooking Time: 5 minutes
Servings: 4

Ingredients:

- Four zucchini, cut into 1/2-inch pieces
- 1 cup of water
- 1/2 tsp. Italian seasoning
- 1/2 tsp. red pepper flakes
- 1 tsp. garlic, minced
- 1 tbsp. olive oil
- 1/2 cup can tomato, crushed
- Salt

Directions

1. Add water and zucchini into the instant pot.
2. Seal pot with lid and cook on high for 2 minutes.
3. Once done, release pressure using quick release. Remove lid.
4. Drain zucchini well and clean the instant pot.
5. Add oil into the inner pot of the instant pot and set the pot on sauté mode.
6. Add garlic and sauté for 30 seconds.
7. Add remaining ingredients and stir well and cook for 2-3 minutes.
8. Serve and enjoy.

Nutrition:
Calories 69
Fat 4.1 g
Carbohydrates 7.9 g
Sugar 3.5 g
Protein 2.7 g

5. Healthy Garlic Eggplant

Preparation Time: 10 minutes
Cooking Time: 10 minutes
Servings: 4

Ingredients:

- One eggplant, cut into 1-inch pieces
- 1/2 cup water
- 1/4 cup can tomato, crushed
- 1/2 tsp. Italian seasoning

- 1 tsp. paprika
- 1/2 tsp. chili powder
- 1 tsp. garlic powder
- 2 tbsp. olive oil
- Salt

Directions

1. Add water and eggplant into the instant pot.
2. Seal pot with lid and cook on high for 5 minutes.
3. Once done, release pressure using quick release. Remove lid.
4. Drain eggplant well and clean the instant pot.
5. Add oil into the inner pot of the instant pot and set the pot on sauté mode.
6. Add eggplant along with remaining ingredients and stir well and cook for 5 minutes.
7. Serve and enjoy.

Nutrition:
Calories 97
Fat 7.5 g
Carbohydrates 8.2 g
Sugar 3.7 g
Protein 1.5 g

6.   Carrot Potato Medley

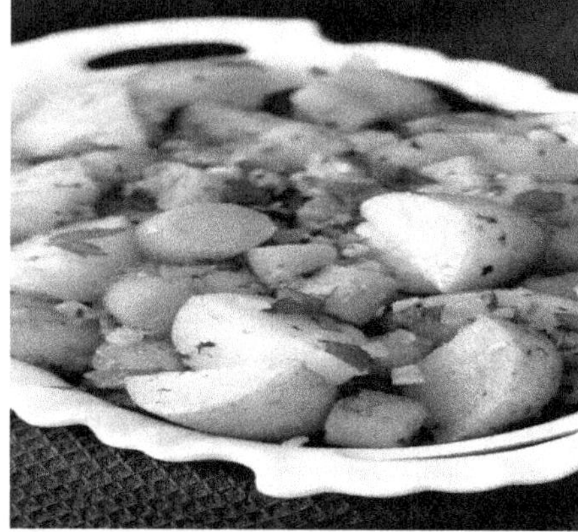

Preparation Time: 10 minutes
Cooking Time: 15 minutes
Servings: 6

Ingredients

- 4 lbs. baby potatoes, clean and cut in half
- 1 1/2 lbs. carrots, cut into chunks
- 1 tsp. Italian seasoning

- 1 1/2 cups vegetable broth
- 1 tbsp. garlic, chopped
- One onion, chopped
- 2 tbsp. olive oil
- Pepper
- Salt

Directions

1. Add oil into the inner pot of the instant pot and set the pot on sauté mode.
2. Add onion and sauté for 5 minutes.
3. Add carrots and cook for 5 minutes.
4. Add remaining ingredients and stir well.
5. Seal pot with lid and cook on high for 5 minutes.
6. Once done, allow to release pressure naturally for 10 minutes, then release remaining using quick release. Remove lid.
7. Stir and serve.

Nutrition:
Calories 283
Fat 5.6 g
Carbohydrates 51.3 g
Protein 10.2 g

7.   Lemon Herb Potatoes

Preparation Time: 10 minutes
Cooking Time: 11 minutes
Servings: 6

Ingredients

- 1 1/2 lbs. baby potatoes, rinsed and pat dry
- 1/2 fresh lemon juice
- 1 tsp. dried oregano
- 1/2 tsp. garlic, minced
- 1 tbsp. olive oil
- 1 cup vegetable broth
- 1/2 tsp. sea salt

Directions:

1. Add broth and potatoes into the instant pot.
2. Seal pot with lid and cook on high for 8 minutes.
3. Once done, release pressure using quick release. Remove lid.

4. Drain potatoes well and clean the instant pot.
5. Add oil into the inner pot of the instant pot and set the pot on sauté mode.
6. Add potatoes, garlic, oregano, lemon juice, and salt and cook for 3 minutes.
7. Serve and enjoy.

Nutrition:
Calories 94
Fat 2.7 g
Carbohydrates 14.6 g
Protein 3.8 g

8. Flavors Basil Lemon Ratatouille

Preparation Time: 10 minutes
Cooking Time: 10 minutes
Servings: 8

Ingredients

- One small eggplant, cut into cubes
- 1 cup fresh basil
- 2 cups grape tomatoes
- One onion, chopped
- Two summer squash, sliced
- Two zucchini, sliced
- 2 tbsp. vinegar
- 2 tbsp. tomato paste
- 1 tbsp. garlic, minced
- One fresh lemon juice
- 1/4 cup olive oil
- Salt

Directions:

1. Add basil, vinegar, tomato paste, garlic, lemon juice, oil, and salt into the blender and blend until smooth.
2. Add eggplant, tomatoes, onion, squash, and zucchini into the instant pot.
3. Pour blended basil mixture over vegetables and stir well.
4. Seal pot with lid and cook on high for 10 minutes.
5. Once done, allow to release pressure naturally. Remove lid.
6. Stir well and serve.

Nutrition:
Calories 103 Fat 6.8 g
Carbohydrates 10.6 g

Sugar 6.1 g
Protein 2.4 g

9. Garlic Basil Zucchini

Preparation Time: 10 minutes
Cooking Time: 8 minutes
Servings: 4

Ingredients

- 14 oz. zucchini, sliced
- 1/4 cup fresh basil, chopped
- 1/2 tsp. red pepper flakes
- 14 oz. can tomatoes, chopped
- 1 tsp. garlic, minced
- 1/2 onion, chopped
- 1/4 cup feta cheese, crumbled
- 1 tbsp. olive oil
- Salt

Directions:

1. Add oil into the inner pot of the instant pot and set the pot on sauté mode.
2. Add onion and garlic and sauté for 2 minutes.
3. Add remaining ingredients except for feta cheese and stir well.
4. Seal pot with lid and cook on high for 6 minutes.
5. Once done, allow to release pressure naturally. Remove lid.
6. Top with feta cheese and serve.

Nutrition:
Calories 99
Fat 5.7 g
Carbohydrates 10.4 g
Sugar 6.1 g
Protein 3.7 g

10. Feta Green Beans

Preparation Time: 10 minutes
Cooking Time: 15 minutes
Servings: 4

Ingredients:

- 1 1/2 lbs. green beans, trimmed
- 1/4 cup feta cheese, crumbled
- 28 oz. can tomatoes, crushed
- 2 tsp. oregano
- 1 tsp. cumin

- 1/2 cup water
- 1 tbsp. olive oil
- 1 tbsp. garlic, minced
- One onion, chopped
- 1 lb. baby potatoes, clean and cut into chunks
- Pepper
- Salt

Directions:

1. Add oil into the inner pot of the instant pot and set the pot on sauté mode.
2. Add onion and garlic and sauté for 3-5 minutes.
3. Add remaining ingredients except for feta cheese and stir well.
4. Seal pot with lid and cook on high for 10 minutes.
5. Once done, allow to release pressure naturally for 5 minutes then release remaining using quick release. Remove lid.
6. Top with feta cheese and serve.

Nutrition:
Calories 234
Fat 6.1 g
Carbohydrates 40.7 g
Protein 9.7 g
Cholesterol 8 mg

11. Garlic Parmesan Artichokes

Preparation Time: 10 minutes
Cooking Time: 10 minutes
Servings: 4

Ingredients:

- Four artichokes, wash, trim, and cut top
- 1/2 cup vegetable broth
- 1/4 cup parmesan cheese, grated
- 1 tbsp. olive oil
- 2 tsp. garlic, minced

Directions

1. Pour broth into the instant pot, then place steamer rack in the pot.
2. Place artichoke steam side down on steamer rack into the pot.

3. Sprinkle garlic and grated cheese on top of artichokes and season with salt. Drizzle oil over artichokes.
4. Seal pot with lid and cook on high for 10 minutes.
5. Once done, release pressure using quick release. Remove lid.
6. Serve and enjoy.

Nutrition:
Calories 132
Fat 5.2 g
Carbohydrates 17.8 g
Protein 7.9 g
Cholesterol 4 mg

12. Delicious Pepper Zucchini

Preparation Time: 10 minutes
Cooking Time: 10 minutes
Servings: 6

Ingredients:

- One zucchini, sliced
- Two poblano peppers, sliced
- 1 tbsp. sour cream
- 1/2 tsp. ground cumin
- One yellow squash, sliced
- 1 tbsp. garlic, minced
- 1/2 onion, sliced
- 1 tbsp. olive oil
- Salt

Directions

1. Add oil into the inner pot of the instant pot and set the pot on sauté mode.
2. Add Poblano peppers and sauté for 5 minutes
3. Add onion and garlic and sauté for 3 minutes.
4. Add remaining ingredients except for sour cream and stir well.
5. Seal pot with lid and cook on high for 2 minutes.
6. Once done, release pressure using quick release. Remove lid.
7. Add sour cream and stir well and serve.

Nutrition:

Calories 42 Fat 2.9 g
Carbohydrates 4 g

Sugar 1.7 g

Protein 1 g

Cholesterol 1 mg

13. Celery Carrot Brown Lentils

Preparation Time: 10 minutes

Cooking Time: 25 minutes

Servings: 6

Ingredients

- 2 cups dry brown lentils, rinsed and drained
- 2 1/2 cups vegetable stock
- Two tomatoes, chopped
- 1/2 tsp. red pepper flakes
- 1/2 tsp. ground cinnamon
- One bay leaf
- 1 tbsp. tomato paste
- Two celery stalks, diced
- Two carrots, grated
- 1 tbsp. garlic, minced
- Two onions, chopped
- 1/4 cup olive oil
- Pepper
- Salt

Directions

1. Add oil into the inner pot of the instant pot and set the pot on sauté mode.
2. Add celery, carrot, garlic, onion, pepper, and salt and sauté for 3 minutes.
3. Add remaining ingredients and stir everything well.
4. Seal pot with lid and cook on high for 22 minutes.
5. Once done, release pressure using quick release. Remove lid.
6. Stir well and serve.

Nutrition:

Calories 137

Fat 8.8 g

Carbohydrates 12.3 g

Protein 3.1 g

14. Lemon Artichokes

Preparation Time: 10 minutes

Cooking Time: 20 minutes

Servings: 4

Ingredients:

- Four artichokes trim and cut the top
- 1/4 cup fresh lemon juice
- 2 cups vegetable stock
- 1 tsp. lemon zest, grated
- Pepper
- Salt

Directions:

1. Pour the stock into the instant pot, then place the steamer rack in the pot.
2. Place artichoke steam side down on steamer rack into the pot.
3. Sprinkle lemon zest over artichokes—season with pepper and salt.
4. Pour lemon juice over artichokes.
5. Seal pot with lid and cook on high for 20 minutes.
6. Once done, allow to release pressure naturally for 5 minutes, then release remaining using quick release. Remove lid.
7. Serve and enjoy.

Nutrition:

Calories 83

Fat 0.4 g

Carbohydrates 17.9 g

Protein 5.6 g

15. Easy Chili Pepper Zucchinis

Preparation Time: 10 minutes

Cooking Time: 10 minutes

Servings: 4

Ingredients

- Four zucchinis, cut into cubes
- 1/2 tsp. red pepper flakes
- 1/2 tsp. cayenne
- 1 tbsp. chili powder
- 1/4 cup vegetable stock
- Salt

Directions:

1. Add all ingredients into the inner pot of the instant pot and stir well.
2. Seal pot with lid and cook on high for 10 minutes.

3. Once done, allow to release pressure naturally for 10 minutes, then release remaining using quick release. Remove lid.
4. Stir and serve.

Nutrition:
Calories 38 Fat 0.7 g
Carbohydrates 8.8 g
Protein 2.7 g

16. Delicious Okra

Preparation Time: 10 minutes
Cooking Time: 10 minutes
Servings: 4

Ingredients:

- 2 cups okra, chopped
- 2 tbsp. fresh dill, chopped
- 1 tbsp. paprika
- 1 cup can tomato, crushed
- Pepper
- Salt

Directions:

1. Add all ingredients into the inner pot of the instant pot and stir well.
2. Seal pot with lid and cook on high for 10 minutes.
3. Once done, allow to release pressure naturally for 5 minutes, then release remaining using quick release. Remove lid.
4. Stir well and serve.

Nutrition:
Calories 37
Fat 0.5 g
Carbohydrates 7.4 g
Protein 2 g

17. Tomato Dill Cauliflower

Preparation Time: 10 minutes
Cooking Time: 12 minutes
Servings: 4

Ingredients:

- 1 lb. cauliflower florets, chopped
- 1 tbsp. fresh dill, chopped
- 1/4 tsp. Italian seasoning

- 1 tbsp. vinegar
- 1 cup can get tomatoes, crushed
- 1 cup vegetable stock
- 1 tsp. garlic, minced
- Pepper
- Salt

Directions:

1. Add all ingredients except dill into the instant pot and stir well.
2. Seal pot with lid and cook on high for 12 minutes.
3. Once done, allow to release pressure naturally for 10 minutes, then release remaining using quick release. Remove lid.
4. Garnish with dill and serve.

Nutrition:
Calories 47
Fat 0.3 g
Carbohydrates 10 g
Protein 3.1 g

18. Parsnips with Eggplant

Preparation Time: 10 minutes
Cooking Time: 12 minutes
Servings: 4

Ingredients

- Two parsnips, sliced
- 1 cup can get tomatoes, crushed
- 1/2 tsp. ground cumin
- 1 tbsp. paprika
- 1 tsp. garlic, minced
- One eggplant, cut into chunks
- 1/4 tsp. dried basil
- Pepper
- Salt

Directions:

1. Add all ingredients into the instant pot and stir well.
2. Seal pot with lid and cook on high for 12 minutes.
3. Once done, release pressure using quick release. Remove lid.
4. Stir and serve.

Nutrition:

Calories 98 0.7 g
Carbohydrates 23 g
Protein 2.8 g

19.   Easy Garlic Beans

Preparation Time: 10 minutes
Cooking Time: 5 minutes
Servings: 4
Ingredients:

- 1 lb. green beans, trimmed
- 1 1/2 cup vegetable stock
- 1 tsp. garlic, minced
- 1 tbsp. olive oil
- Pepper
- Salt

Directions:

1. Add all ingredients into the instant pot and stir well.
2. Seal pot with lid and cook on high for 5 minutes.
3. Once done, release pressure using quick release. Remove lid.
4. Stir and serve.

Nutrition:

Calories 69
Fat 3.7 g
Carbohydrates 8.7 g
Sugar 1.9 g
Protein 2.3 g

20.   Vegan Carrots & Broccoli

Preparation Time: 10 minutes
Cooking Time: 5 minutes
Servings: 6
Ingredients:

- 4 cups broccoli florets
- Two carrots, peeled and sliced
- 1/4 cup water
- 1/2 lemon juice
- 1 tsp. garlic, minced
- 1 tbsp. olive oil
- 1/4 cup vegetable stock
- 1/4 tsp. Italian seasoning
- Salt

Directions:

1. Add oil into the inner pot of the instant pot and set the pot on sauté mode.
2. Add garlic and sauté for 30 seconds.
3. Add carrots and broccoli and cook for 2 minutes.
4. Add remaining ingredients and stir everything well.
5. Seal pot with lid and cook on high for 3 minutes.
6. Once done, release pressure using quick release. Remove lid.
7. Stir well and serve.

Nutrition:

Calories 51 Fat 2.6 g
Carbohydrates 6.3 g
Sugar 2.2 g
Protein 2 g

21.   Rosemary-Roasted   Red Potatoes

Preparation Time: 5 minutes
Cooking Time: 20 minutes
Servings: 6

Ingredients:

- 1 pound red potatoes, quartered
- ¼ cup olive oil
- ½ tsp. kosher salt
- ¼ tsp. black pepper
- One garlic clove, minced
- Four rosemary sprigs

Directions:

1. Preheat the air fryer to 360°F.
2. In a large bowl, toss the potatoes with olive oil, salt, pepper, and garlic until well coated.
3. Pour the potatoes into the air fryer basket and top with the sprigs of rosemary.
4. Roast for 10 minutes, then stir or toss the potatoes and roast for 10 minutes more.
5. Remove the rosemary sprigs and serve the potatoes. Season with additional salt and pepper, if needed.

Nutrition:

Calories: 133
Fat: 9g
Protein: 1g
Carbohydrates: 12g

22. Roasted Radishes with Sea Salt

Preparation Time: 5 minutes
Cooking Time: 18 minutes
Servings: 4
Prep Time: 5 minutes
Cook Time: 18 minutes

Ingredients:

- 1 pound radishes, ends trimmed if needed
- 2 tbsp. olive oil
- ½ tsp. sea salt

Directions:

1. Preheat the air fryer to 360°F.
2. In a large bowl, combine the radishes with olive oil and sea salt.
3. Pour the radishes into the air fryer and cook for 10 minutes. Stir or turn the radishes over and cook for 8 minutes more, then serve.

Nutrition:
Calories: 78 Fat: 9g
Protein: 1g Carbohydrates: 4g Fiber: 2g

23. Garlic Zucchini and Red Peppers

Preparation Time: 5 minutes
Cooking Time: 15 minutes
Servings: 6

Ingredients:

- Two medium zucchini, cubed
- One red bell pepper, diced
- Two garlic cloves, sliced
- 2 tbsp. olive oil
- ½ tsp. salt

Directions:

1. Preheat the air fryer to 380°F.
2. In a large bowl, mix the zucchini, bell pepper, and garlic with olive oil and salt.
3. Pour the mixture into the air fryer basket, and roast for 7 minutes. Shake or stir, then burn for 7 to 8 minutes more.

Nutrition:
Calories: 60 Fat: 5g
Protein: 1g Carbohydrates: 4g
Fiber: 1g

24. Parmesan and Herb Sweet Potatoes

Preparation Time: 10 minutes
Cooking Time: 18 minutes
Servings: 4

Ingredients:

- Two large sweet potatoes, peeled and cubed
- ¼ cup olive oil
- 1 tsp. dried rosemary
- ½ tsp. salt
- 2 tbsp. shredded Parmesan

Directions:

1. Preheat the air fryer to 360°F.
2. In a large bowl, toss the sweet potatoes with olive oil, rosemary, and salt.
3. Pour the potatoes into the air fryer basket and roast for 10 minutes, then stir the potatoes and sprinkle the Parmesan over the top. Continue roasting for 8 minutes more.
4. Serve hot and enjoy.

Nutrition:
Calories: 186
Fat: 14g
Protein: 2g
Carbohydrates: 13g
Fiber: 2g

25. Roasted Brussels sprouts with Orange and Garlic

Preparation Time: 5 minutes
Cooking Time: 10 minutes
Servings: 4

Ingredients:

- 1 pound Brussels sprouts, quartered
- Two garlic cloves, minced
- 2 tbsp. olive oil
- ½ tsp. salt
- One orange, cut into rings

Directions:

1. Preheat the air fryer to 360°F.
2. In a large bowl, toss the quartered Brussels sprouts with garlic, olive oil, and salt until well coated.
3. Pour the Brussels sprouts into the air fryer, lay the orange slices on top of them, and roast for 10 minutes.
4. Remove from the air fryer and set the orange slices aside. Toss the Brussels sprouts before serving.

Nutrition:
Calories: 111
Fat: 7g
Protein: 4g
Carbohydrates: 11g
Fiber: 4g

26. Crispy Lemon Artichoke Hearts

Preparation Time: 10 minutes
Cooking Time: 15 minutes
Servings: 2
Ingredients:

- 1 (15-ounce) can artichoke hearts in water, drained
- One egg
- 1 tbsp. water
- ¼ cup whole wheat bread crumbs
- ¼ tsp. salt
- ¼ tsp. paprika
- ½ lemon

Directions:

1. Preheat the air fryer to 380°F.
2. In a medium shallow bowl, beat together the egg and water until frothy.
3. In a separate medium shallow bowl, mix the bread crumbs, salt, and paprika.
4. Dip each artichoke heart into the egg mixture, then into the bread crumb mixture, coating the outside with the crumbs. Place the artichokes hearts in a single layer of the air fryer basket.
5. Fry the artichoke hearts for 15 minutes.
6. Remove the artichokes from the air fryer, and squeeze fresh lemon juice over the top before serving.

Nutrition:
Calories: 91 Fat: 2g
Protein: 5g
Carbohydrates: 16g
Fiber: 8g

27. Citrus Green Beans with Red Onions

Preparation Time: 5 minutes
Cooking Time: 10 minutes
Servings: 6

Ingredients:

- 1 pound fresh green beans, trimmed
- ½ red onion, sliced
- 2 tbsp. olive oil
- ½ tsp. salt
- ¼ tsp. black pepper
- 1 tbsp. lemon juice
- Lemon wedges, for serving

Directions:

1. Preheat the air fryer to 360°F. In a large bowl, toss the green beans, onion, olive oil, salt, pepper, and lemon juice until combined.
2. Pour the mixture into the air fryer and roast for 5 minutes. Stir well and roast for 5 minutes more.
3. Serve with lemon wedges.

Nutrition:
Calories: 67
Fat: 5g
Protein: 1g
Carbohydrates: 6g
Fiber: 2g

28. Spiced Honey-Walnut Carrots

Preparation Time: 5 minutes
Cooking Time: 12 minutes
Servings: 6
Ingredients:

- 1 pound baby carrots
- 2 tbsp. olive oil
- ¼ cup raw honey
- ¼ tsp. ground cinnamon
- ¼ cup black walnuts, chopped

Directions:

1. Preheat the air fryer to 360°F.
2. In a large bowl, toss the baby carrots with olive oil, honey, and cinnamon until well coated.
3. Pour into the air fryer and roast for 6 minutes. Shake the basket, sprinkle the walnuts on top, and roast for 6 minutes more.
4. Remove the carrots from the air fryer and serve.

Nutrition:

Calories: 146

Fat: 8g

Protein: 1g

Carbohydrates: 20g

Fiber: 3g

29. Roasted Grape Tomatoes and Asparagus

Preparation Time: 5 minutes

Cooking Time: 12 minutes

Servings: 6

Ingredients:

- 2 cups grape tomatoes
- One bunch of asparagus, trimmed
- 2 tbsp. olive oil
- Three garlic cloves, minced
- ½ tsp. kosher salt

Directions:

1. Preheat the air fryer to 380°F.
2. In a large bowl, combine all of the ingredients, tossing until the vegetables are well coated with oil.
3. Pour the vegetable mixture into the air fryer basket and spread into a single layer, then roast for 12 minutes.

Nutrition:

Calories: 57

Fat: 5g

Protein: 1g

Carbohydrates: 4g

Fiber: 1g

30. Stuffed Red Peppers with Herbed Ricotta and Tomatoes

Preparation Time: 10 minutes

Cooking Time: 20 minutes

Servings: 4

Ingredients:

- Two red bell peppers
- 1 cup cooked brown rice
- 2 Roma tomatoes, diced
- One garlic clove, minced
- ¼ tsp. salt
- ¼ tsp. black pepper
- 4 ounces ricotta
- 3 tbsp. fresh basil, chopped
- 3 tbsp. fresh oregano, chopped
- ¼ cup shredded Parmesan, for topping

Directions:

1. Preheat the air fryer to 360°F.
2. Cut the bell peppers in half and remove the seeds and stem.
3. In a medium bowl, combine the brown rice, tomatoes, garlic, salt, and pepper.
4. Distribute the rice filling evenly among the four bell pepper halves.
5. In a small bowl, combine the ricotta, basil, and oregano. Put the herbed cheese over the top of the rice mixture in each bell pepper.
6. Place the bell peppers into the air fryer and roast for 20 minutes.
7. Remove and serve with shredded Parmesan on top.

Nutrition:

Calories: 156

Fat: 6g

Protein: 8g

Carbohydrates: 19g

Fiber: 3g

31. Easy Greek Briami (Ratatouille)

Preparation Time: 15 minutes

Cooking Time: 40 minutes

Servings: 6

Ingredients:

- Two russet potatoes, cubed
- ½ cup Roma tomatoes, cubed
- One eggplant, cubed

- One zucchini, cubed
- One red onion, chopped
- One red bell pepper, chopped
- Two garlic cloves, minced
- 1 tsp. dried mint
- 1 tsp. dried parsley
- 1 tsp. dried oregano
- ½ tsp. salt
- ½ tsp. black pepper
- ¼ tsp. red pepper flakes
- 1/3 cup olive oil
- 1 (8-ounce) can tomato paste
- ¼ cup vegetable broth
- ¼ cup water

Directions:

1. Preheat the air fryer to 320°F.
2. In a large bowl, combine the potatoes, tomatoes, eggplant, zucchini, onion, bell pepper, garlic, mint, parsley, oregano, salt, black pepper, and red pepper flakes.
3. In a small bowl, mix the olive oil, tomato paste, broth, and water.
4. Pour the oil-and-tomato-paste mixture over the vegetables and toss until everything is coated.
5. Pour the coated vegetables into the air fryer basket in an even layer and roast for 20 minutes. After 20 minutes, stir well and spread out again. Roast for an additional 10 minutes, then repeat the process and cook for another 10 minutes.

Nutrition:
Calories: 280
Fat: 13g
Protein: 6g
Carbohydrates: 40g

32. Parmesan-Thyme Butternut Squash

Preparation Time: 15 minutes
Cooking Time: 20 minutes
Servings: 4

Ingredients:

- 2 ½ cups butternut squash, cubed into 1-inch pieces (approximately one medium)
- 2 tbsp. olive oil
- ¼ tsp. salt
- ¼ tsp. garlic powder
- ¼ tsp. black pepper
- 1 tbsp. fresh thyme
- ¼ cup grated Parmesan

Directions:

1. Preheat the air fryer to 360°F.
2. In a large bowl, combine the cubed squash with olive oil, salt, garlic powder, pepper, and thyme until the squash is well coated.
3. Pour this mixture into the air fryer basket, and roast for 10 minutes. Stir and roast another 8 to 10 minutes more.
4. Remove the squash from the air fryer and toss with freshly grated Parmesan before serving.

Nutrition:
Calories: 127
Fat: 9g
Protein: 3g
Carbohydrates: 11g
Fiber: 2g

33. Zucchini Tomato Potato Ratatouille

Preparation Time: 10 minutes
Cooking Time: 10 minutes
Servings: 6

Ingredients

- 1 1/2 lbs. potatoes, cut into cubes
- 1/2 cup fresh basil
- 28 oz. fire-roasted tomatoes, chopped
- One onion, chopped
- Four mushrooms, sliced
- One bell pepper, diced
- 12 oz. eggplant, diced
- 8 oz. zucchini, diced
- 8 oz. yellow squash, diced
- Pepper
- Salt

Directions:

1. Add all ingredients except basil into the instant pot and stir well.
2. Seal pot with lid and cook on high for 10 minutes.
3. Once done, release pressure using quick release. Remove lid.
4. Add basil and stir well and serve.

Nutrition:

Calories: 149 kcal

Protein: 6.05 g

Fat: 0.88 g

Carbohydrates: 32.49 g

34. Crispy Garlic Sliced Eggplant

Preparation Time: 5 minutes

Cooking Time: 25 minutes

Servings: 4

Ingredients:

- One egg
- 1 tbsp. water
- ½ cup whole wheat bread crumbs
- 1 tsp. Garlic powder
- ½ tsp. Dried oregano
- ½ tsp. Salt
- ½ tsp. paprika
- One medium eggplant, sliced into ¼-inch-thick rounds
- 1 tbsp. olive oil

Directions:

1. Preheat the air fryer to 360°F.
2. In a medium shallow bowl, beat together the egg and water until frothy.
3. In a separate medium shallow bowl, mix bread crumbs, garlic powder, oregano, salt, and paprika.
4. Dip each eggplant slice into the egg mixture, then into the bread crumb mixture, coating the outside with crumbs. Place the pieces in a single layer in the bottom of the air fryer basket.
5. Drizzle the tops of the eggplant slices with the olive oil, then fry for 15 minutes. Turn each piece and cook for an additional 10 minutes.

Nutrition:

Calories: 137

Fat: 5g

Protein: 5g

Carbohydrates: 19g

Fiber: 5g

35. Dill-and-Garlic Beets

Preparation Time: 10 minutes

Cooking Time: 30 minutes

Servings: 4

Ingredients:

- Four beets, cleaned, peeled, and sliced
- One garlic clove, minced
- 2 tbsp. chopped fresh dill
- ¼ tsp. salt
- ¼ tsp. black pepper
- 3 tbsp. olive oil

Directions:

1. Preheat the air fryer to 380°F.
2. In a large bowl, mix all of the ingredients, so the beets are well coated with the oil.
3. Pour the beet mixture into the air fryer basket, and roast for 15 minutes before stirring, then continue roasting for 15 minutes more.

Nutrition:

Calories: 126

Fat: 10g

Protein: 1g

Carbohydrates: 8g

Fiber: 2g

36. Citrus-Roasted Broccoli Florets

Preparation Time: 5 minutes

Cooking Time: 12 minutes

Servings: 6

Ingredients:

- 4 cups broccoli florets (approximately one large head)
- 2 tbsp. olive oil
- ½ tsp. salt
- ½ cup orange juice
- 1 tbsp. raw honey
- Orange wedges, for serving (optional)

Directions:
1. Preheat the air fryer to 360°F.
2. In a large bowl, combine the broccoli, olive oil, salt, orange juice, and honey. Toss the broccoli in the liquid until well coated.
3. Pour the broccoli mixture into the air fryer basket and cook for 6 minutes. Stir and cook for 6 minutes more.
4. Serve alone or with orange wedges for additional citrus flavor, if desired.

Nutrition:
Calories: 80
Fat: 5g
Protein: 2g
Carbohydrates: 9g
Fiber: 2g

~ 143 ~

CHAPTER 10:

Desserts

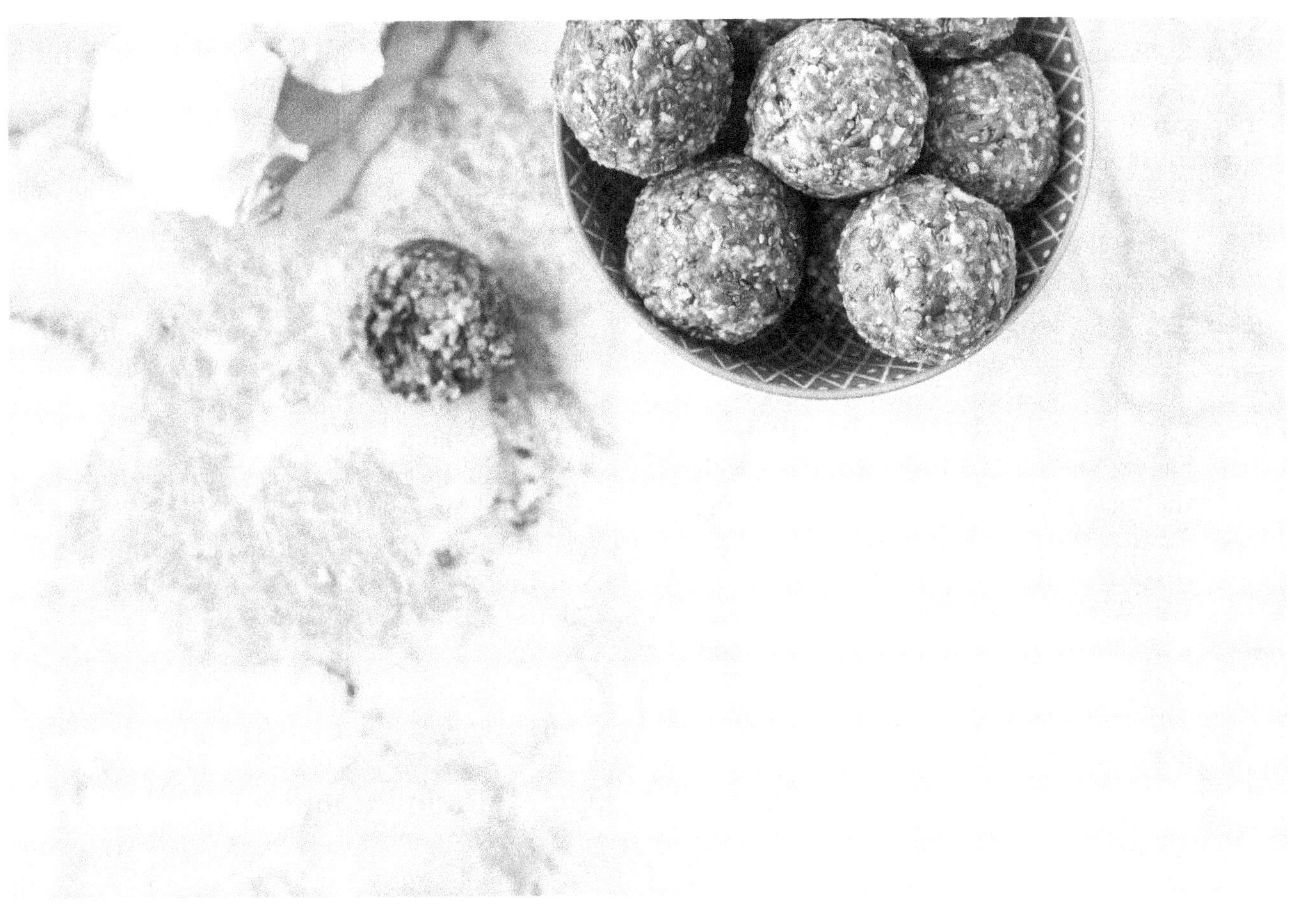

1. Mascarpone and Fig Crostini

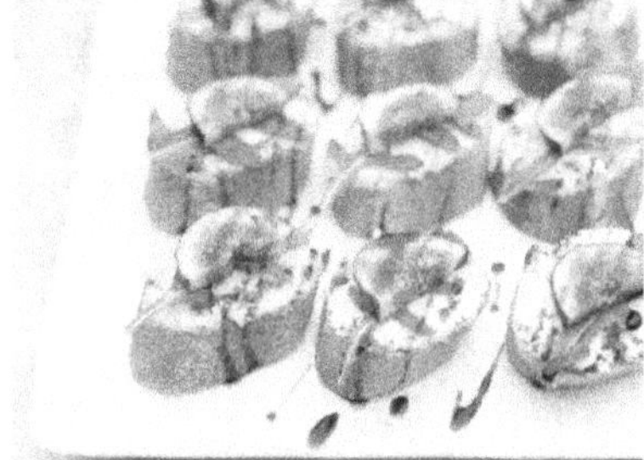

Preparation Time: 10 minutes
Cooking Time: 10 minutes
Servings: 6-8
Ingredients: One long French baguette

- 4 tbsp. (½ stick) salted butter, melted
- 1 (8-ounce) tub mascarpone cheese
- 1 (12-ounce) jar fig jam or preserves

Directions:

1. Preheat the oven to 350°F.
2. Slice the bread into ¼-inch-thick slices.
3. Layout the sliced bread on a single baking sheet and brush each slice with the melted butter. Put the single baking sheet in the oven and toast the bread for 5 to 7 minutes until golden brown.
4. Let the bread cool slightly. Spread it with a tsp. or so of the mascarpone cheese on each piece of the bread.
5. Top with a tsp. or so of the jam. Serve immediately.

Nutrition: Calories: 445 Fat: 24g Carbs: 48g Protein: 3g

2. Crunchy Sesame Cookies

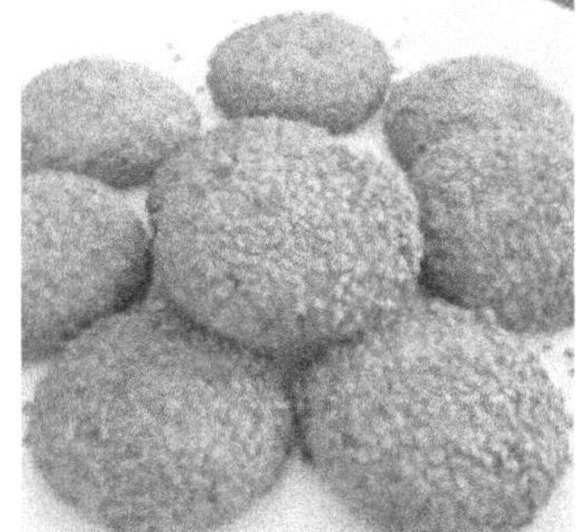

Preparation Time: 10 minutes
Cooking Time: 15 minutes
Servings: 14-16

Ingredients:

- 1 cup sesame seeds, hulled
- 1 cup sugar
- 8 tbsp. (1 stick) salted butter softened
- Two large eggs
- 1¼ cups flour

Directions:

1. Preheat the oven to 350°F. Toast the sesame seeds on a baking sheet for 3 minutes. Set aside and leave to cool.
2. Using a mixer, cream together the sugar and butter.
3. Put the eggs in one at a time until well-blended.
4. Add the flour and toasted sesame seeds and mix until well-blended.
5. Drop spoonful of cookie dough onto a baking sheet and form them into round balls, about 1-inch in diameter, similar to a walnut.
6. Put in the oven and bake for 5 to 7 minutes or until golden brown.
7. Let the cookies cool and enjoy.

Nutrition:
Calories: 218
Fat: 12g
Carbs: 25g
Protein: 4g

3. Almond Cookies

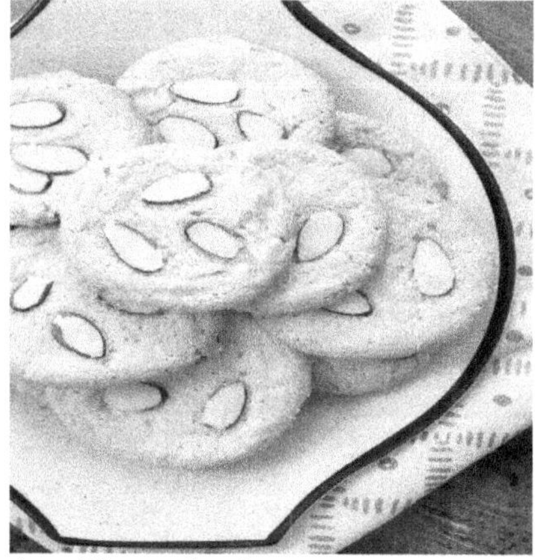

Preparation Time: 5 minutes
Cooking Time: 10 minutes
Servings: 4-6
Ingredients:

- ½ cup sugar

- 8 tbsp. (1 stick) room temperature salted butter
- One large egg
- 1½ cups all-purpose flour
- 1 cup ground almonds or almond flour

Directions:

1. Preheat the oven to 375°F.
2. Using a mixer, cream together the sugar and butter.
3. Add the egg and mix until combined.
4. Alternately add the flour and ground almonds, ½ cup at a time, while the mixer is slow.
5. Once everything is combined, line a baking sheet with parchment paper. Drop a tbsp. Of dough on the baking sheet, keeping the cookies at least 2 inches apart.
6. Put the single baking sheet in the oven and bake just until the cookies start to turn brown around the edges for about 5 to 7 minutes.

Nutrition:

Calories: 604
Fat: 36g
Carbs: 63g
Protein: 11g

4.   Baklava and Honey

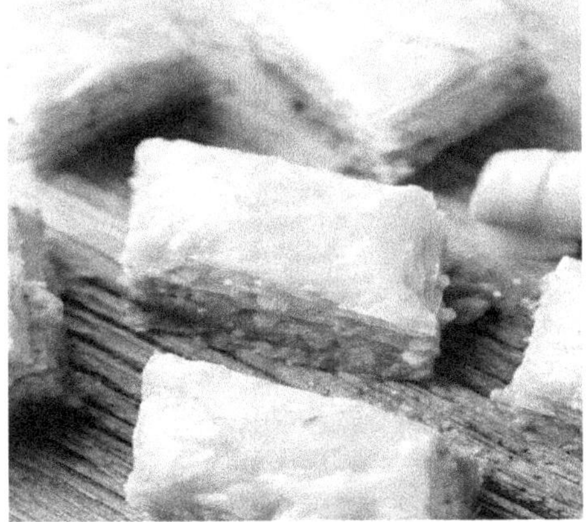

Preparation Time: 40 minutes
Cooking Time: 1 hour
Servings: 6-8

Ingredients:

- 2 cups chopped walnuts or pecans
- 1 tsp. cinnamon
- 1 cup of melted unsalted butter
- 1 (16-ounce) package phyllo dough, thawed
- 1 (12-ounce) jar honey

Directions:

1. Preheat the oven to 350°F.
2. In a bowl, combine the chopped nuts and cinnamon.
3. Using a brush, butter the sides and bottom of a 9-by-13-inch baking dish.
4. Take off the phyllo dough from the package and cut it to the baking dish's size using a sharp knife.
5. Put one sheet of phyllo dough on the bottom of the dish, brush with butter, and repeat until you have eight layers.
6. Sprinkle 1/3 cup of the nut mixture over the phyllo layers. Top with a sheet of phyllo dough, butter that sheet, and repeat until you have four sheets of buttered phyllo dough.
7. Sprinkle 1/3 cup of the nut mixture for another layer of nuts. Repeat the layering of nuts and four sheets of buttered phyllo until all the nut mixture is gone. The last layer should be eight buttered sheets of phyllo.
8. Before you bake, cut the baklava into desired shapes; traditionally, this is diamonds, triangles, or squares.
9. Bake the baklava for about 1 hour just until the top layer is golden brown.
10. While the baklava is baking, heat the honey in a pan just until it is warm and comfortable to pour.
11. Once the baklava is done baking, pour the honey evenly over the baklava and let it absorb it, about 20 minutes. Serve warm or at room temperature.

Nutrition:

Calories: 1235
Fat: 89g
Carbs: 109g
Protein: 18g

5. Mango Snow

Preparation Time: 5 minutes
Cooking Time: 2 hours
Servings: 8

Ingredients:

- 4 cups frozen mango in pieces
- One can of condensed milk (14 ounces/396 g)
- One can of evaporated milk (12 ounces /340 g)
- Mint leaves (decoration)
- Cookies (decoration)

Directions:

1. Blend the mango, the condensed milk, and the evaporated milk at high speed for 5 minutes.
2. Transfer the mixture to the mixing bowl. Cover and leave to cool for at least 2 hours in the freezer.
3. Garnish with mint leaves and cookies.

Nutrition:
Calories: 411 Carbohydrates: 84g
Protein: 1g Fat: 8g

6. Minty Coconut Cream

Preparation Time: 4 minutes
Cooking Time: 0 minutes
Servings: 2

Ingredients:

- One banana, peeled
- 2 cups coconut flesh, shredded
- 3 tbsp. mint, chopped
- One and ½ cups coconut water
- 2 tbsp. stevia
- ½ avocado pitted and peeled

Directions:

1. In a blender, combine the coconut with the banana and the rest of the ingredients, pulse well, divide into cups and serve cold.

Nutrition:
Calories 193
Fat: 5.4g
Fiber: 3.4g
Carbs: 7.6g

Protein: 3g

7. Watermelon Cream

Preparation Time: 15 minutes
Cooking Time: 0 minutes
Servings: 2

Ingredients:

- 1-pound watermelon, peeled and chopped
- 1 tsp. vanilla extract
- 1 cup heavy cream
- 1 tsp. lime juice
- 2 tbsp. stevia

Directions:

1. In a blender, combine the watermelon with the cream and the rest of the ingredients, pulse well, divide into cups and keep in the fridge for 15 minutes before serving.

Nutrition:
Calories 122
Fat: 5.7g
Fiber: 3.2g
Carbs: 5.3g
Protein: 0.4g

8. Grap Stew

Preparation Time: 10 minutes
Cooking Time: 10 minutes
Servings: 4

Ingredients:

- 2/3 cup stevia
- 1 tbsp. olive oil
- 1/3 cup coconut water
- 1 tsp. vanilla extract
- 1 tsp. lemon zest, grated
- 2 cup red grapes, halved

Directions:

1. Heat a pan with the water over medium heat, add the oil, stevia, and the rest of the ingredients, toss, simmer for 10 minutes, divide into cups, and serve.

Nutrition:
Calories: 122
Fat: 3.7g
Fiber: 1.2g
Carbs: 2.3g

Protein: 0.4g

9. Cocoa Sweet Cherry Cream

Preparation Time: 2 hours
Cooking Time: 0 minutes
Servings: 4

Ingredients:

- ½ cup cocoa powder
- ¾ cup red cherry jam
- ¼ cup stevia
- 2 cups water
- 1-pound cherries pitted and halved

Directions:

1. In a blender, mix the cherries with the water and the rest of the ingredients, pulse well, divide into cups, and keep in the fridge for 2 hours before serving.

Nutrition:
Calories: 162
Fat: 3.4g
Fiber: 2.4g
Carbs: 5g
Protein: 1g

10. Banana Dessert with Chocolate Chips

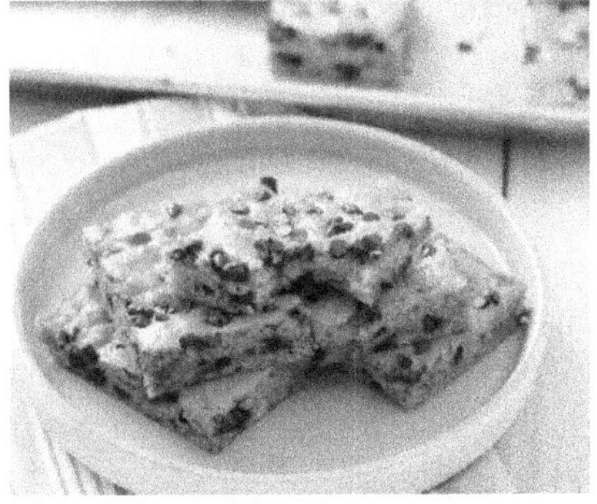

Preparation Time: 20 minutes
Cooking Time: 30 minutes
Servings: 24

Ingredients:

- 2/3 c. white sugar
- ¾ c. butter
- 2/3 c. brown sugar
- One egg, beaten
- 1 tsp. vanilla extract
- 1 c. banana puree
- One ¾ c. flour
- 2 tsp. Baking powder
- ½ tsp. salt
- 1 c. semi-sweet chocolate chips

Directions:

1. Preheat oven to 350°F
2. In a bowl, add the sugars and butter and beat until lightly colored
3. Add the egg and vanilla.
4. Add the banana puree and stir
5. In another bowl, mix baking powder, flour, and salt. Add this mixture to the butter mixture
6. Stir in the chocolate chips
7. Prepare a baking pan and place the dough onto it
8. Bake for 20 minutes and let it cool for 5 minutes before slicing into equal squares

Nutrition:
Calories 174
Fat 8.2g
Carbs 25.2g
Protein 1.7g

11. Cranberry and Pistachio Biscotti

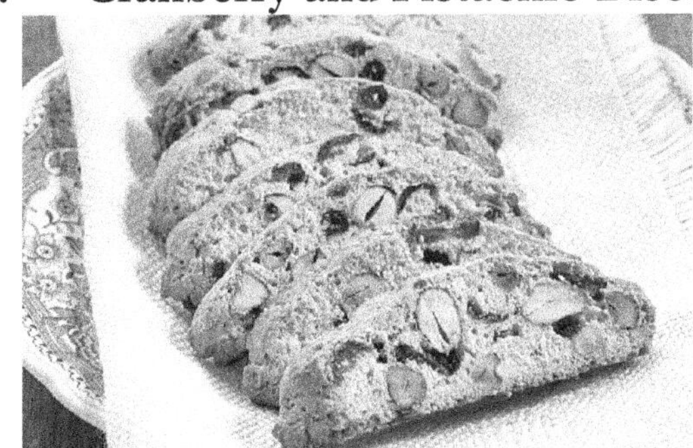

Preparation Time: 20 minutes
Cooking Time: 60 minutes
Servings: 4

Ingredients:

- ¼ c. light olive oil
- ¾ c. white sugar
- 2 tsp. Vanilla extract
- ½ tsp. almond extract
- Two eggs
- One ¾ c. all-purpose flour
- ¼ tsp. salt
- 1 tsp. baking powder

- ½ c. dried cranberries
- 1 ½ c. pistachio nuts

Directions:

1. Preheat the oven at 300 F/ 148 C
2. Combine olive oil and sugar in a bowl and mix well
3. Add eggs, almond, and vanilla extracts, stir
4. Add baking powder, salt, and flour
5. Add cranberries and nuts, mix
6. Divide the dough in half — form two 12 x 2-inch logs on a parchment baking sheet.
7. Set in the oven and bake for 35 minutes or until the blocks are golden brown. Set from range and allow cooling for about 10 minutes.
8. Set the oven to 275 F/ 135 C
9. Cut diagonal trunks into 3/4-inch-thick slices. Place on the sides on the baking sheet covered with parchment
10. Bake for about 8 - 10 minutes or until dry
11. You can serve it both hot and cold

Nutrition:

Calories 92
Fat 4.3g
Carbs 11.7g
Protein 2.1g

12.   Minty Watermelon Salad

Preparation Time: 10 minutes
Cooking Time: 0 minutes
Servings: 6-8
Ingredients:

- One medium watermelon
- 1 cup fresh blueberries
- 2 tbsp. fresh mint leaves
- 2 tbsp. lemon juice
- 1/3 cup honey

Directions:

1. Cut the watermelon into 1-inch cubes. Put them in a bowl.
2. Evenly distribute the blueberries over the watermelon.
3. Chop the mint leaves and then put them into a separate bowl.
4. Add the lemon juice and honey to the mint and whisk together.
5. Drizzle the mint dressing over the watermelon and blueberries. Serve cold

Nutrition:
Calories 238
Fat 1g
Carbs 61g
Protein 4g

13.   Date and Nut Balls

Preparation Time: 10 minutes
Cooking Time: 10 minutes
Servings: 6-8

Ingredients:

- 1 cup walnuts or pistachios
- 1 cup unsweetened shredded coconut
- 14 Medjool dates, pits removed
- 8 tbsp. (1 stick) butter, melted

Directions:

1. Preheat the oven to 350°F.
2. Put the nuts on a baking sheet. Toast the nuts for 5 minutes.
3. Put the shredded coconut on a clean baking sheet; toast just until it turns golden brown, about 3 to 5 minutes (coconut burns fast, so keep an eye on it). Once done, remove it from the oven and put it in a shallow bowl.
4. Inside a food processor with a chopping blade put the nuts until they have a medium chop. Put the chopped nuts into a medium bowl.
5. Add the dates and melted butter to the food processor and blend until the dates become a thick paste. Pour the chopped nuts into the food processor with the dates and pulse until the mixture is combined, about 5 to 7 pulses.
6. Remove the mixture from the food processor and scrape it into a large bowl.
7. To make the balls, spoon 1 to 2 tbsp. of the date mixture into the palm of your hand and roll around between your hands until you form a ball. Put the ball

on a clean, lined baking sheet. Repeat this until all of the mixtures are formed into balls.

8. Roll each ball in the toasted coconut until the outside of the ball is coated, put the ball back on the baking sheet, and repeat.

9. Put all the balls into the fridge for 20 minutes before serving so that they firm up. You can also store any leftovers inside the refrigerator in an airtight container.

Nutrition:

Calories 489

Fat 35g

Carbs 48g

Protein 5g

14.   Creamy Rice Pudding

Preparation Time: 5 minutes

Cooking Time: 45 minutes

Servings: 6

Ingredients:

- 1¼ cups long-grain rice
- 5 cups whole milk
- 1 cup sugar
- 1 tbsp. of rose water/orange blossom water
- 1 tsp. cinnamon

Directions:

1. Rinse the rice under cold water for 30 seconds.

2. Add the rice, milk, and sugar to a large pot. Bring to a gentle boil while continually stirring.

3. Lessen the heat to low and then let simmer for 40 to 45 minutes, stirring every 3 to 4 minutes so that the rice does not stick to the bottom of the pot.

4. Add the rosewater at the end and simmer for 5 minutes.

5. Divide the pudding into six bowls. Sprinkle the top with cinnamon. Let it cool for over an hour before serving. Store in the fridge.

Nutrition:

Calories 394

Fat 7g

Carbs 75g

Protein 9g

15.   Ricotta-Lemon Cheesecake

Preparation Time: 5 minutes

Cooking Time: 1 hour

Servings: 8-10

Ingredients:

- 2 (8-ounce) packages full-fat cream cheese
- 1 (16-ounce) container full-fat ricotta cheese
- 1½ cups granulated sugar
- 1 tbsp. lemon zest
- 5 large eggs
- Nonstick cooking spray

Directions:

1. Preheat the oven to 350°F.

2. Blend the cream cheese and ricotta cheese.

3. Blend in the sugar and lemon zest.

4. Blend in the eggs; drop in 1 egg at a time, blend for 10 seconds, and repeat.

5. Put a 9-inch spring form pan with parchment paper and nonstick spray. Wrap the bottom of the pan with foil. Pour the cheesecake batter into the pan.

6. To make a water bath, get a baking or roasting pan larger than the cheesecake pan. Fill the roasting pan about 1/3 of the way up with warm water. Put the cheesecake pan into the water bath. Put the whole thing in the oven and let the cheesecake bake for 1 hour.

7. After baking is complete, remove the cheesecake pan from the water bath and remove the foil. Let the cheesecake cool for 1 hour on the countertop. Then put it in the fridge to cool for at least 3 hours before serving.

Nutrition:

Calories 489

Fat 31g

Carbs 42g

Protein 15g

16.   Blueberry-Blackberry Ice Pops

Preparation Time: 5 minutes + 2 hours to freeze
Cooking Time: 0 minutes
Servings: 2
Ingredients:

- ½ (13.5-ounce) can coconut cream,
- ¾ cup unsweetened full-fat coconut milk, or ¾ cup heavy (whipping) cream
- 2 tsp. Swerve natural sweetener or 2 drops liquid stevia
- ½ tsp. vanilla extract
- ¼ cup mixed blueberries and blackberries

Directions:

1. Add together the coconut cream, sweetener, and vanilla.
2. Add the mixed berries, and then pulse just a few times.
3. Pour it into ice pop molds and freeze for at least about 2 hours before serving.

Nutrition:
Calories: 165
Carbohydrates: 4g
Protein: 1g
Fat: 17g

17.   Strawberry-Lime Ice Pops

Preparation Time: 5 minutes + 2 hours to freeze
Cooking Time: 0 minutes
Servings: 4
Ingredients:

- ½ (13.5-ounce) can coconut cream,
- ¾ cup unsweetened full-fat coconut milk
- or ¾ cup heavy (whipping) cream
- 2 tsp. Swerve natural sweetener or two drops of liquid stevia
- 1 tbsp. freshly squeezed lime juice
- ¼ cup hulled and sliced strawberries (fresh or frozen)

Directions:

1. Mix the coconut cream, sweetener, and lime juice in a blend
2. Add the strawberries, and pulse just a few times, so the strawberries retain their texture.

3. Pour into ice pop molds, and freeze for at least 2 hours before serving.

Nutrition:
Calories: 166
Carbohydrates: 5g
Protein: 1g
Fat: 17g

18.   Chocolate Lava Cake

Preparation Time: 30 minutes
Cooking Time: 3 hours
Servings: 12
Ingredients:

- 1 ½ c. stevia sweetener, divided
- ½ c. almond flour
- 5 tbsps. Unsweetened cocoa powder
- ½ tsp. salt
- 1 tsp. baking powder
- Three whole eggs
- Three egg yolks
- ½ c. butter, melted
- 1 tsp. vanilla extract
- 2 c. hot water
- 4 ounces' sugar-free chocolate chips

Directions:

1. Grease the inside of the Crockpot.
2. In a bowl, mix the stevia sweetener, almond flour, cocoa powder, salt, and baking powder.
3. In another bowl, mix the eggs, egg yolks, butter, and vanilla extract. Pour in hot water.
4. Pour the wet ingredients into the dry ingredients and fold to create a batter.
5. Add the chocolate chips last
6. Pour into the greased Crockpot and cook on low for 3 hours.
7. Allow cooling before serving.

Nutrition:
Calories: 157
Carbohydrates: 5.5g
Protein: 10.6g
Fat: 13g

19.   Lemon and Watermelon Granita

Preparation Time: 10 minutes + 3 hours to freeze

Cooking Time: 0 minutes

Servings: 4

Ingredients:

- 4 cups watermelon cubes
- ¼ cup honey
- ¼ cup freshly squeezed lemon juice

Directions:

1. In a blender, combine the watermelon, honey, and lemon juice. Purée all the ingredients, then pour into a 9-by-9-by-2-inch baking pan and place in the freezer.
2. Every 30 to 60 minutes, run a fork across the frozen surface to fluff and create ice flakes. Freeze for about 3 hours total and serve.

Nutrition:

Calories: 153

Carbohydrates: 39g

Protein: 2g

Fat: 1g

20.   Baked Apples with Walnuts and Spices

Preparation Time: 10 minutes

Cooking Time: 45 minutes

Servings: 4

Ingredients:

- Four apples
- ¼ cup chopped walnuts
- 2 tbsp. honey
- 1 tsp. ground cinnamon
- ¼ tsp. ground nutmeg
- ¼ tsp. ground ginger
- Pinch sea salt

Directions:

1. Preheat the oven to 375°F.
2. Cut the tops off the apples and then use a metal spoon or a paring knife to remove the cores, leaving the bottoms of the apples intact. Place the apples cut-side up in a 9-by-9-inch baking pan.
3. Stir together the walnuts, honey, cinnamon, nutmeg, ginger, and sea salt. Put the mixture into the centers of the apples. Bake the apples for about 45 minutes until browned, soft, and fragrant. Serve warm.

Nutrition:

Calories: 199

Carbohydrates: 41g

Protein: 5g

Fat: 5g

21.   Vanilla Pudding with Strawberries

Preparation Time: 10 minutes

Cooking Time: 10 minutes + chilling time

Servings: 4

Ingredients:

- 2¼ cups skim milk, divided
- One egg, beaten
- ½ cup sugar
- 1 tsp. vanilla extract
- Pinch sea salt
- 3 tbsp. cornstarch
- 2 cups sliced strawberries

Directions:

1. In a small bowl, whisk 2 cups of milk with the egg, sugar, vanilla, and sea salt. Transfer the mixture to a medium pot, place it over medium heat, and slowly bring to a boil, whisking constantly.
2. Whisk the cornstarch with ¼ cup of milk. In a thin stream, whisk this slurry into the boiling mixture in the pot. Cook until it thickens, stirring constantly. Boil for 1 minute more, stirring constantly.
3. Spoon the pudding into four dishes and refrigerate to chill. Serve topped with the sliced strawberries.

Nutrition:

Calories: 209

Carbohydrates: 43g

Protein: 6g

Fat: 1g

22.   Mixed Berry Frozen Yogurt Bar

Preparation Time: 10 minutes
Cooking Time: 0 minutes
Servings: 8

Ingredients:

- 8 cups low-fat vanilla frozen yogurt (or flavor of choice)
- 1 cup sliced fresh strawberries
- 1 cup fresh blueberries
- 1 cup fresh blackberries
- 1 cup fresh raspberries
- ½ cup chopped walnuts

Directions:

1. Apportion the yogurt among eight dessert bowls.
2. Serve the toppings family-style, and let your guests choose their toppings and spoon them over the yogurt.

Nutrition:
Calories: 81 Carbohydrates: 9g Protein: 3g Fat: 5g

23.   Cherry Brownies with Walnuts

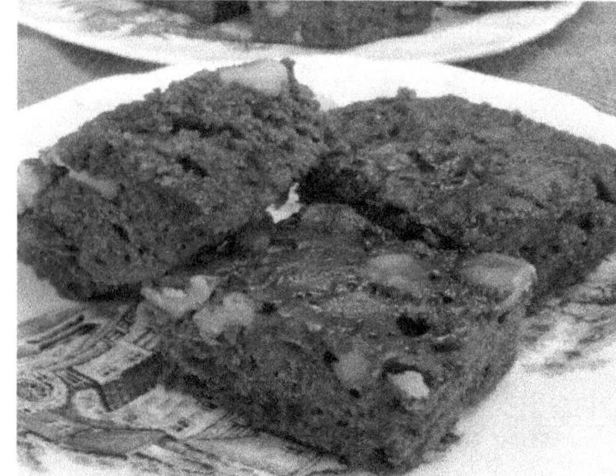

Preparation Time: 10 minutes
Cooking Time: 25-30 minutes
Servings: 9

Ingredients:

- Nine fresh cherries that are stemmed and pitted or nine frozen cherries
- ½ cup sugar or sweetener substitute
- ¼ cup extra virgin olive oil
- 1 tsp. vanilla extract
- ¼ tsp. sea salt
- ½ cup whole-wheat pastry flour
- ¼ tsp. baking powder
- 1/3 cup walnuts, chopped
- Two eggs
- ½ cup plain Greek yogurt
- 1/3 cup cocoa powder, unsweetened

Directions:

1. Make sure one of the metal racks in your oven is set in the middle.
2. Turn the temperature on your oven to 375 degrees Fahrenheit.
3. Using cooking spray, grease a 9-inch square pan.
4. Take a large bowl and add the oil and sugar or sweetener substitute. Whisk the ingredients well.
5. Add the eggs and use a mixer to beat the ingredients together.
6. Pour in the yogurt and continue to beat the mixture until it is smooth.
7. Take a medium bowl and combine the cocoa powder, flour, sea salt, and baking powder by whisking them together.
8. Combine the powdered ingredients into the wet ingredients and use your electronic mixer to thoroughly incorporate the ingredients together.
9. Add in the walnuts and stir.
10. Pour the mixture into the pan.
11. Sprinkle the cherries on top and push them into the batter. You can use any design, but it is best to make three rows and three columns with the cherries. This ensures that each piece of the brownie will have one cherry.
12. Put the batter into the oven and turn your timer to 20 minutes.
13. Check that the brownies are done using the toothpick test before removing them from the oven. Push the toothpick into the middle of the brownies and once it comes out clean, remove the brownies.
14. Let the brownies cool for 5 to 10 minutes before cutting and serving.

Nutrition:
Calories: 225 Fats: 10 grams
Carbohydrates: 30 grams

Protein: 5 grams.

24.   Fruit Dip

Preparation Time: 10 minutes
Cooking Time: 10-15 minutes
Servings: 10
Ingredients:

- ¼ cup coconut milk, full-fat is best
- ¼ cup vanilla yogurt
- 1/3 cup marshmallow creme
- 1 cup cream cheese, set at room temperature
- 2 tbsp. maraschino cherry juice

Directions:

1. In a large bowl, add the coconut milk, vanilla yogurt, marshmallow creme, cream cheese, and cherry juice.
2. Using an electric mixer, set to low speed and blend the ingredients until the fruit dip is smooth.
3. Serve the dip with some of your favorite fruits, and enjoy!

Nutrition:
Calories: 110
Fats: 11 grams
Carbohydrate 3 grams
Protein: 3 grams.

25.   A Lemony Treat

Preparation Time: 20 minutes
Cooking Time: 30 minutes
Servings: 4

Ingredients:

- One lemon, medium in size
- 1 ½ tsp. cornstarch
- 1 cup Greek yogurt, plain is best
- Fresh fruit
- ¼ cup cold water
- 2/3 cup heavy whipped cream
- 3 tbsp. honey
- Optional: mint leaves

Directions:

1. Take a large glass bowl and your metal electric mixer and set them in the refrigerator so they can chill.
2. In a separate bowl, add the yogurt and set that in the fridge.
3. Zest the lemon into a medium microwavable bowl.
4. Cut the lemon in half and then squeeze 1 tbsp. of lemon juice into the bowl.
5. Combine the cornstarch and water. Mix the ingredients thoroughly.
6. Pour in the honey and whisk the ingredients together.
7. Put the mixture into the microwave for 1 minute on high.
8. Once the microwave stops, remove the mixture and stir.
9. Set it back into the microwave for 15 to 30 seconds or until the mixture starts to bubble and thicken.
10. Take the bowl of yogurt from the fridge and pour in the warm mixture while whisking.
11. Put the yogurt mixture back into the fridge.
12. Take the large bowl and beaters out of the fridge.
13. Put your electronic mixer together and pour the whipped cream into the chilled bowl.
14. Beat the cream until soft peaks start to form. This can take up to 3 minutes, depending on how fresh your cream is.
15. Remove the yogurt from the fridge.
16. Fold the yogurt into the cream using a rubber spatula. Remember to lift and turn the mixture, so it doesn't deflate.
17. Place back into the fridge until you are serving the dessert or for 15 minutes. The dessert should not be in the refrigerator for longer than 1 hour.
18. When you serve the lemony goodness, you will spoon it into four dessert dishes and drizzle with extra honey or even melt some chocolate to drizzle on top.
19. Add a little fresh mint and enjoy!

Nutrition:

Calories: 241
Fats: 16 grams
Carbohydrates: 21 grams
Protein: 7 grams

26. Melon with Ginger

Preparation Time: 10 minutes
Cooking Time: 10-15 minutes
Servings: 4

Ingredients:

1. ½ cantaloupe, cut into 1-inch chunks
2. 2 cups of watermelon, cut into 1-inch chunks
3. 2 cups honeydew melon, cut into 1-inch chunks
4. 2 tbsp. of raw honey
5. Ginger, 2 inches in size, peeled, grated, and preserve the juice
6. Directions:
7. In a large bowl, combine your cantaloupe, honeydew melon, and watermelon. Gently mix the ingredients.
8. Combine the ginger juice and stir.
9. Drizzle on the honey, serve, and enjoy! You can also chill the mixture for up to an hour before serving.

Nutrition:
Calories: 91
Fats: 0 grams
Carbohydrates: 23 grams
Protein: 1 gram

27. Almond Shortbread Cookies

Preparation Time: 15 minutes
Cooking Time: 25 minutes
Servings: 16

Ingredients:

- ½ cup coconut oil
- 1 tsp. vanilla extract
- 2 egg yolks
- 1 tbsp. brandy
- 1 cup powdered sugar
- 1 cup finely ground almonds
- 3 ½ cups cake flour
- ½ cup almond butter
- 1 tbsp. water or rose flower water

Directions:

1. In a large bowl, combine the coconut oil, powdered sugar, and butter. If the butter is not soft, you want to wait until it softens up. Use an electric mixer to beat the ingredients together at high speed.
2. In a small bowl, add the egg yolks, brandy, water, and vanilla extract. Whisk well.
3. Fold the egg yolk mixture into the large bowl.
4. Add the flour and almonds. Fold and mix with a wooden spoon.
5. Place the mixture into the fridge for at least 1 hour and 30 minutes.
6. Preheat your oven to 325 degrees Fahrenheit.
7. Take the mixture, which now looks like dough, and divide it into 1-inch balls.
8. With a piece of parchment paper on a baking sheet, arrange the cookies and flatten them with a fork or your fingers.
9. Place the cookies in the oven for 13 minutes, but watch them, so they don't burn.
10. Transfer the cookies onto a rack to cool for a couple of minutes before enjoying!

Nutrition:
Calories: 250
Fats: 14 grams
Carbohydrates: 30 grams
Protein: 3 grams.

28. Chocolate Fruit Kebabs

Preparation Time: 10 minutes
Cooking Time: 30 minutes
Servings: 6

Ingredients:

- 24 blueberries
- 12 strawberries with the green leafy top part removed
- 12 green or red grapes, seedless
- 12 pitted cherries
- 8 ounces chocolate

Directions:

1. Line a baking sheet with a piece of parchment paper and place 6 -inch long wooden skewers on top of the paper.
2. Start by threading a piece of fruit onto the skewers. You can create and follow any pattern that you like with the ingredients. An example pattern is one strawberry, one cherry, blueberries, two grapes. Repeat the pattern until all of the fruit is on the skewers.
3. In a saucepan on medium heat, melt the chocolate. Stir continuously until the chocolate has melted completely.
4. Carefully scoop the chocolate into a plastic sandwich bag and twist the bag closed, starting right above the chocolate.
5. Snip the corner of the bag with scissors.
6. Drizzle the chocolate onto the kebabs by squeezing it out of the bag.
7. Put the baking pan into the freezer for 20 minutes.
8. Serve and enjoy!

Nutrition:

Calories: 254

Fats: 15 grams

Carbohydrates: 28 grams

Protein: 4 grams.

29. Mediterranean Blackberry Ice Cream

Preparation Time: 10 minutes

Cooking Time: 15 minutes

Servings: 6

Ingredients:

- Three egg yolks
- One container of Greek yogurt
- 1 pound mashed blackberries
- ½ tsp. vanilla essence
- 1 tsp. arrowroot powder
- ¼ tsp. ground cloves
- 5 ounces sugar or sweetener substitute
- 1 pound heavy cream

Directions:

1. In a small bowl, add the arrowroot powder and egg yolks. Whisk or beat them with an electronic mixture until they are well combined.
2. Set a saucepan on top of your stove and turn your heat to medium.
3. Add the heavy cream and bring it to a boil.
4. Turn off the heat and add the egg mixture into the cream through folding.
5. Turn the heat back on to medium and pour in the sugar. Cook the mixture for 10 minutes or until it starts to thicken.
6. Remove the mixture from heat and place it in the fridge so it can completely cool. This should take about one hour.
7. Once the mixture is cooled, add in the Greek yogurt, ground cloves, blackberries, and vanilla by folding in the ingredients.
8. Transfer the ice cream into a container and place it in the freezer for at least two hours.
9. Serve and enjoy!

Nutrition:

Calories: 402

Fats: 20 grams

Carbohydrate 52 grams

Protein: 8 grams.

30 Day Meal Plan

Days	Breakfast	Lunch	Dinner	Snacks
1	Banana Nut Oatmeal	Mediterranean Spaghetti	Chicken Wrap	Walnuts Yogurt Dip
2	Greek Yogurt Pancakes	Chicken With Peas	Rosemary-Roasted Red Potatoes	Creamy Pepper Spread
3	Omelet Provencale	Caprese Pasta Salad	Lemon Herb Potatoes	Perfect Queso
4	Chili Cheese Omelet	Sautéed Cabbage With Parsley	Almond Chicken Bites	Fluffy Bites
5	Strawberry Marmalade	Mushroom And Garlic Spaghetti	Baked Salmon With Tarragon Mustard Sauce	Coconut Fudge
6	Avocado Breakfast Sandwiches	Greek Green Beans	Baked Lemon Salmon	Tasty Black Bean Dip
7	Greek Yogurt Parfait	One-Pan Tuscan Chicken	Baby Kale And Cabbage Salad	Cucumber Tomato Okra Salsa
8	Yogurt Cheese	Tomato Pasta Fagioli	Chicken And Black Beans	Cheesy Corn Dip
9	Arugula Frittata	Delicious Pepper Zucchini	Halibut And Quinoa Mix	Chili Mango And Watermelon Salsa
10	Sweet Oatmeal	Celery Carrot Brown Lentils	Lemon and Dates Barramundi	Yogurt Dip
11	Avocado Toast	Catfish Fillets And Rice	Halibut And Quinoa Mix	Slow-Cooked Cheesy Artichoke Dip
12	Baked Eggs With Parsley	Pasta With Creamy Sauce	Butter Chicken Thighs	cucumber sandwich bites
13	Yogurt With Dates	Feta Macaroni	Parmesan Chicken	Rosemary Hummus
14	Artichoke Omelet	Pecan Salmon Fillets	Turkey And Cranberry Sauce	Sausage Queso Dip
15	Banana Oats	Salmon and Broccoli	Parmesan-Thyme Butternut Squash	Yogurt Dip
16	Sun-Dried Tomatoes Oatmeal	Turkey Burgers With Mango Salsa	Cod and Mushrooms Mix	Nutmeg Nougat
17	Berry Oats	Crispy Garlic Sliced Eggplant	Chicken and Olives Salsa	Sweet Almond Bites
18	Greek Yogurt Parfait	Basil Buckwheat Pasta	Chili Chicken Mix	Walnuts Yogurt Dip
19	Banana Quinoa	Parmesan and Herb Sweet Potatoes	Salmon And Peach Pan	Flavorful Italian Peppers
20	Greek Yogurt W/Berries & Seeds	Crispy Lemon Artichoke Hearts	Garlic Zucchini And Red Peppers	Cheese Stuff Artichokes

21	Mediterranean Diet Breakfast Tostadas	Citrus Green Beans With Red Onions	Feta Green Beans	Walnuts Yogurt Dip
22	Greek Yogurt W/Berries & Seeds	Sesame Shrimp Mix	Healthy Vegetable Medley	Flavorful Roasted Baby Potatoes
23	Yogurt Cheese	Baked Shrimp Mix	Flavors Basil Lemon Ratatouille	Cucumber Rolls
24	Chickpea Soup With Shrimp	Shrimp And Lemon Sauce	Garlic Basil Zucchini	Olives And Cheese Stuffed Tomatoes
25	Creamy Loaded Mashed Potatoes	Cauliflower Rice	Baked Halibut Steaks With Vegetables	Mixed Berry Frozen Yogurt Bar
26	Mediterranean Egg Scramble	Bacon Linguine Pasta	Turkey, Artichokes and Asparagus	Veggie Fritters
27	Avocado Green Apple Breakfast Smoothie	Tomato Dill Cauliflower	Double Cheesy Bacon Chicken	Wrapped Plums
28	Breakfast Toast	Parsnips With Eggplant	Crispy Italian Chicken	Bulgur Lamb Meatballs
29	Savory Egg Galettes	Halibut Roulade	Olive Oil Poached Cod	Almond Shortbread Cookies
30	Spinach Frittata	Chicken And Butter Sauce	Pistachio-Crusted Halibut	Crunchy Sesame Cookies

Conclusion:

Thank you for reading the Mediterranean Diet cookbook. This book's recipes and ideas will benefit you and your family. The Mediterranean diet is well-known for its heart-health benefits. The secret to a balanced diet is variety. Every day, eat a variety of foods from different food classes. Every day, make half of your grain products whole grain. Per day, consume at least three servings of vegetables and fruits, as well as two servings of milk. Good fats are included in many of the recipes in this book to help reduce bad cholesterol and avoid heart attacks. Some of the recipes may have more calories than other diet meals, but these healthy oils may help you reduce your cholesterol. Your body will benefit from Greek yogurt's mucus-relief properties. Avocados, for example, are high in healthy fats. Avocados have more beneficial fats than any other vegetable. To get the correct amount of healthy fats, the recipes in this book only use one-third of an avocado. In addition to regulating insulin levels, the Mediterranean diet helps to normalize blood sugar levels. This is the secret to eating well. Your body will be in a safe condition for the remainder of your life if you can keep your blood sugar in check.

The Mediterranean diet reduces the consumption of refined foods. It's been associated with a lower risk of experiencing a variety of chronic diseases, including obesity, diabetes, coronary artery disease, and cognitive impairment, both of which are included among these advantages. The Mediterranean diet is known for its heavily spiced dishes that require little to no preparation. They are usually made from fresh ingredients obtained from the outdoors, such as nuts, fruits, vegetables, and fish. Another important feature of the diet that contributes to body alkalinity is the use of alkaline foods such as vegetables and herbs for seasoning. Any individuals who have tried the Mediterranean diet have had promising effects in terms of weight loss. A decrease of body weight, as well as the loss of abdominal skin and a reduction of blood pressure, are among the promising outcomes.

When you adopt a Mediterranean diet, your body adapts to a long-term model of calorie burning. The absorption of carbohydrates in foods is greatly reduced as you consume foods and beverages that contain more natural oils. You'll also eat meals that are lower in fat, which is healthier for the body's absorption of nutrients. This diet can be used effectively by people who do not have glucose resistance issues. One of the best things about this diet is that it includes fruit, fish, and vegetables in addition to meat. Meat makes up just about a portion of the Mediterranean diet. Reduced abdominal weight, heartbeat irregularities, and blood sugar levels are only a few of the advantages of this diet. Moving on, it's easy to see that a Mediterranean diet will be beneficial to many people's health.

The most significant advantage of making a comprehensive lifestyle improvement is that it will immediately increase your physical health and well-being. Â Apart from the healing effects, you would also benefit from the life-extension aspect. As a result of the advantages it has, it is becoming increasingly attractive to many people. It is one of the best diets for preventing cardiovascular disease. It contains a lot of nuts and has a lot of anti-inflammatory properties that favor people who consume Mediterranean foods.

www.ingramcontent.com/pod-product-compliance
Lightning Source LLC
Chambersburg PA
CBHW080024260726
48658CB00007B/2451